The Prevention of FOOD POISONING

3rd edition (Revised)

Jill Trickett MSc

Formerly Senior Lecturer in Food Hygiene
Salford College of Technology

Stanley Thornes (Publishers) Ltd

First published in 1978 by:
Stanley Thornes (Publishers) Ltd
Ellenborough House
Wellington Street
CHELTENHAM GL50 1YW

Second edition 1986
Third edition 1992
Revised third edition 1996

96   97   98   99   00   /   10   9   8   7   6   5   4   3   2   1

A catalogue record for this book is available from the British Library.
ISBN 0 7487 1522 3

Text set in 11/13 pt Italia by Tech-Set, Gateshead, Tyne and Wear.
Printed and bound in Great Britain at Redwood Books, Trowbridge, Wiltshire.

Contents

Preface to the third edition

My aim in writing this book is quite simply to provide an introduction to the subject of food poisoning. The fact that the number of outbreaks of food poisoning is increasing each year despite apparently higher living standards and high standards of personal hygiene suggests that many staff employed in the catering industry, and many housewives, have no knowledge of the causes and prevention of food poisoning.

The book seeks to offer an interesting and logical approach to the basic principles of bacterial growth with special emphasis on pathogenic bacteria, their sources, means of access to the kitchen, ways of controlling their growth in foods and hence the prevention of food poisoning. No previous knowledge of the subject is required but for anyone already acquainted with the basic ideas, the provision of sub-headings should make it possible to refer to any particular subject area.

This new edition includes a summary of the main provisions of the latest food hygiene legislation and a new chapter on food preservation. There are extensions to some chapters and many minor amendments have been made but the basic structure remains the same.

The book covers the syllabuses of The Royal Institute of Public Health and Hygiene Certificate in Food Hygiene and the Handling of Food, and The Institute of Environmental Health Officers' Intermediate Food Hygiene Certificate. It provides a good groundwork for more advanced examinations but remains a readable text for those who are not taking examinations but merely wish to understand the principles of the prevention of food poisoning.

J. Trickett   November 1991

Acknowledgements

My sincere thanks go to: Mr R. R. Charnock of The College, Swindon who first suggested that I should write this book; and to him and Mrs B. D. Martin who read the manuscript making a number of suggestions.

Mr D. Harley and Mr B. Mallett of the Public Health Laboratory, Southampton General Hospital for preparing slides and to the Department of Teaching Media, Southampton General Hospital who prepared the photographs.

Dr A. C. Buck, consultant pathologist, Princess Margaret Hospital, Swindon for providing further slides.

Mr R. Moore, formerly Superintendent Food Safety and Hygiene Officer, Sheffield, and Mr M. S. Wildsmith, senior Public Health Inspector, Thamesdown for their help with technical data.

My parents for checking through the manuscript, and Mrs W. E. Greenway for typing it.

I am grateful for the help received from Rentokil Ltd (photographs on pages 98, 99, 101, 102), Clenaglass Electric Ltd (reference for illustration on page 87), Haigh Engineering Ltd, Pifco Ltd, Sissons of Sheffield (reference for illustration on page 94), Public Health Laboratory, Withington Hospital (pages 20, 25, 29 and 34), and Miss M. A. Munford of Marks and Spencer PLC whilst putting together the second edition. Thanks are due to The Community Disease Surveillance Centre for permission to use their figures and to The Health Education Council for permission to reproduce their posters; also to Dr Helen Whitwell for her help with photographs and to my husband Stuart for his help in many ways.

Thanks are due for permission to reproduce questions from past examination papers to the Royal Society of Health, the Associated Examining Board, the University of London Examining Board and the Joint Matriculation Board.

Cover illustrations: Anthony Blake Photo Library, London School of Hygiene and Tropical Medicine and Science Photo Library, Dr Tony Brain and Science Photo Library, and Mr T. Moran.

Chapter 1

Introduction to Bacteria

Bacteria are so small that they can be seen only through a microscope. A bacterium has a very simple structure consisting of one cell only whereas the human body (or that of any animal or insect) is made up of countless numbers of different cells.

Approximately one million bacteria clumped together would cover a pin-head. There are many different types of bacteria and they vary in shape and size but the ones found in food are usually spherical (*cocci*), rod-shaped (*bacilli*) or comma-shaped (*vibrios*).

COCCUS
A spherical or near
spherical cell

BACILLUS
A rod shaped cell — longer
than it is broad

VIBRIO
Curved rods — shaped as
'commas'

Bacteria are present almost everywhere: in the air, on our skin and hair, in our noses and mouths, in our intestinal tracts, in our food, on kitchen equipment, in garden soil and in water. Some are mobile and can swim around in liquids but most cannot move by themselves. These are only transferred by direct contact.

GROWTH AND MULTIPLICATION

If bacteria are supplied with food, water and a warm temperature, they will grow and reproduce by a process known as binary fission. The bacterial cell grows to a maximum size by absorbing simple substances from its environment and then splits into two new identical cells. In

1

optimum conditions (the very best conditions) for growth (see Chapter 2) bacteria will divide into two approximately every twenty minutes.

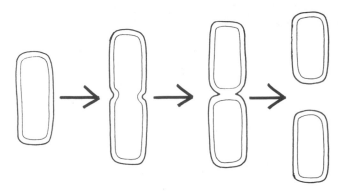

Bacteria reproduce by a process known as binary fission

One bacterium will therefore produce two bacteria after twenty minutes. These two bacteria will then both grow and divide into two after a further twenty minutes making a total of four bacteria after forty minutes. After sixty minutes there will be eight bacteria and after five or six hours there will be thousands of bacteria.

Study the following table to see how quickly the number of bacteria in food can increase. Can you fill in the spaces?

	20 min	40 min	60 min
0 hours	2	4	8
1 hour	16	32	64
2 hours	128	256	
3 hours	1024	2048	4096
4 hours		16 384	
5 hours	65 536		262 144

After six hours in optimum conditions it is possible for one bacterium to become 262 144 bacteria. These bacteria will continue to grow at the same rate until food or an essential growth factor is no longer available or until the presence of poisonous waste products inhibits their growth.

PATHOGENS

Only a few of the thousands of different types of bacteria are responsible for causing illness. Those which do are known as pathogens.
Certain pathogens can make food poisonous by growing and multiplying in it and must normally be present in large numbers in order to
cause illness. Small numbers of most types of pathogenic bacteria can
be swallowed with food without causing any ill effects. However, food
can contain large numbers of food poisoning bacteria and yet look,
smell and taste perfectly wholesome.

SPOILAGE BACTERIA

Certain bacteria are capable of spoiling food without making it
poisonous. The change in odour, taste and appearance of pasteurised
milk on keeping is due to acids produced by bacteria as they grow in
the milk. Meat and fish start to smell and become slimy due to the waste
products of the bacteria that are growing on them. Spoilage bacteria are
not usually pathogenic. However, if food has been kept in conditions
which allow the multiplication of spoilage bacteria, any food poisoning
bacteria which are also present are likely to have had chance to multiply.

USEFUL BACTERIA

Many bacteria perform useful functions and are essential for certain
processes, for example:

1. The manufacture of cheese and yoghurt.

2. The production of some antibiotics and some vitamins.

3. The production of manure from decaying vegetable matter.

YEASTS AND MOULDS

Micro-organisms are living things which are individually too small to be
seen without a microscope. There are many different types. The ones
most frequently found in food, apart from bacteria, are yeasts and
moulds.

Yeasts do not cause food poisoning but some types are capable of
causing food spoilage. They usually spoil acid foods with a high sugar

content, e.g. fruit juices, yoghurts, wines. One type of yeast has great commercial importance because it is used for the production of bread and alcohol (beer, wine and cider).

Moulds do not normally cause food poisoning although some of them can produce mycotoxins (poisonous substances). Moulds present in grain or nuts which are stored in damp conditions produce mycotoxins which may cause cancer. Food is frequently spoiled by moulds, particularly fairly dry or acid food. Black or blue-green moulds are a familiar sight on bread and citrus fruits. Some moulds are used in the production of antibiotics and blue cheeses.

SUMMARY

1. Bacteria are very small and can only be seen with a microscope.

2. In optimum conditions for growth, bacteria will divide into two approximately every twenty minutes.

3. There are thousands of different types of bacteria but only a few of them can cause food poisoning.

4. Bacteria, yeasts and moulds are all micro-organisms which are frequently present in food.

Chapter 2

The Growth Requirements of Food Poisoning Bacteria

In order to grow and multiply, bacteria require four things: warmth, food, moisture and time.

WARMTH

The bacteria which cause food poisoning prefer to live at the temperature of the human body, 37 °C, and it is at this temperature that they will grow and multiply at the fastest rate. As the temperature increases from 37 °C to 63 °C the rate of growth slows down and at temperatures above this bacteria will gradually be killed. The length of time and the temperature required to kill them will depend on the type of bacteria and the food involved. They are normally killed in 1–2 minutes in boiling water, unless they are able to form spores (see p. 8).

If the temperature of the food is decreased from 37 °C to 5 °C the bacteria will continue to multiply but the rate of multiplication will slow down as the temperature decreases. Bacteria are not killed by low temperatures but they are dormant. This means that they stay alive but stop growing and multiplying. Most food poisoning bacteria will not grow at the temperature of the domestic refrigerator, 1–4 °C, but some spoilage bacteria are able to grow and multiply slowly. When the foods are removed from the refrigerator and warmed up, the rate of bacterial growth increases. Pathogenic and spoilage bacteria remain dormant even in frozen food, but as soon as the food is thawed they will start to grow and multiply again.

In the summer, the temperature in a badly ventilated kitchen can reach 30 °C, which is a temperature at which bacteria can multiply very rapidly. For this reason foods should not be allowed to stand for any length of time in a kitchen. Any preparation should be done as quickly as possible and then the food should be stored in a refrigerator until it is ready to be served.

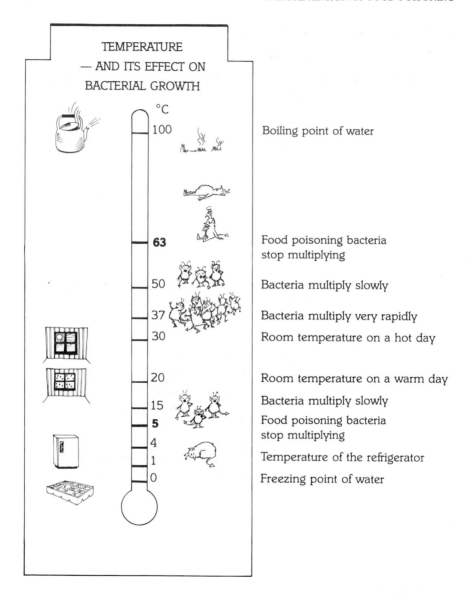

TEMPERATURE
— AND ITS EFFECT ON
BACTERIAL GROWTH

°C

100   Boiling point of water

63   Food poisoning bacteria
             stop multiplying

50   Bacteria multiply slowly

37   Bacteria multiply very rapidly

30   Room temperature on a hot day

20   Room temperature on a warm day

15   Bacteria multiply slowly

5   Food poisoning bacteria
             stop multiplying

4   Temperature of the refrigerator

1

0   Freezing point of water

FOOD

Like all living things bacteria need food. They will live and multiply in many foodstuffs, particularly those which are high in protein and moisture. The foods that we eat that most frequently support bacterial growth are:

1.   Meats, poultry and meat products (meat pies and pasties, sausages).

2. Stocks, gravies, stews and sauces.

3. Milk, cream and egg products (custards, trifles).

The following foods do not normally support the growth of food poisoning bacteria:

1. Acid foods (pickles, citrus fruits).

2. Foods with a high concentration of salt (salted meats, anchovies, olives).

3. Foods with a high concentration of sugar (jams, syrups).

4. Fatty foods (butter, cooking oil).

5. Dry foods (biscuits, flour).

Although bacteria thrive on foods enjoyed by humans, a crumb lodged in a crack on a table or a smear of blood on an unwashed chopping board is sufficient food for thousands of bacteria.

Some of the foods which support bacterial growth

MOISTURE

Like all living things bacteria require moisture for growth. Most foods contain sufficient water for bacterial growth but dehydrated products such as milk powder, dried soup powder and dried egg powder will not allow the growth of bacteria. In dried products bacteria survive but remain dormant until the powders are reconstituted. If a pint of milk is made up from milk powder, it must be stored in a refrigerator as soon as the water is added, to prevent any bacteria present from multiplying.

TIME

If bacteria are provided with food, water and a temperature near 37 °C, they will divide into two every twenty minutes. A few bacteria cannot cause illness but if food contaminated with bacteria is kept for a sufficiently long time in the right conditions the number of bacteria will increase, making the food poisonous. If food is eaten shortly after it is cooked or prepared, the risk of food poisoning is considerably reduced.

AEROBES AND ANAEROBES

Bacteria differ from one another in their requirements for oxygen. Many of them require the presence of air to grow and multiply and these are called aerobes. Some will not multiply in the presence of oxygen and these are called obligate anaerobes. Some can multiply equally well in the presence or absence of oxygen and these are called facultative anaerobes.

SPORES

When bacteria are growing and multiplying we say they are in the vegetative state. In this state they are fairly easily destroyed by heat or chemicals. Some bacteria, but not all, can exist in another form — the spore form. A spore is a rounded body which forms inside the bacterial cell when conditions become unfavourable for growth or multiplication. The rest of the cell then gradually disintegrates leaving only the spore. This spore can resist very high temperatures and high concentrations of chemicals that would kill bacteria in the vegetative state. They can survive at least four hours in boiling water and so they are not destroyed by normal cooking methods. Spores are also formed when there is insufficient moisture present. They can survive for years without food or water, but when conditions again become favourable the spores return to the vegetative state and continue to grow and multiply.

SUMMARY

1. The four requirements for bacterial growth are warmth, food, moisture and time.

2. The bacteria which cause food poisoning grow best at 37 °C.

3. The temperature and humidity of the kitchen provide excellent conditions for the growth and multiplication of bacteria.

4. Bacteria are not killed by the cold but most of those which cause food poisoning stop multiplying in a refrigerator.

5. Bacteria grow best in foods which are high in moisture and are not too acid, not too sugary and not too salty.

6. Bacteria cannot grow and multiply without moisture but they can remain dormant in dried foods.

7. Bacteria in the vegetative state are killed after two minutes in boiling water.

8. Some bacteria form spores which are only destroyed after several hours in boiling water.

Chapter 3

What is Food Poisoning?

Food poisoning is an illness brought about by eating harmful food. The symptoms are usually vomiting, diarrhoea and abdominal pains. Vomiting and diarrhoea are the body's method of disposing of harmful substances from the digestive tract thus preventing them from getting into the blood stream. In a few types of food poisoning the poisons enter the blood stream, causing illness in the body generally, with a wide variety of symptoms.

CAUSES OF FOOD POISONING

The causes of food poisoning fall into four main categories.

1. Bacterial food poisoning The vast majority of all food poisoning cases are caused by bacteria. The food is poisonous because it has been contaminated by pathogenic bacteria which have been allowed to multiply during incorrect storage of the food.

2. Viral food poisoning Certain viruses that cause vomiting and diarrhoea can be transmitted by water and food (see page 125). Viruses require living tissue for growth and therefore will not multiply in the food. The food is merely a means of transport into the human body. They are destroyed by the temperatures reached in normal cooking methods and so viral food poisoning is usually transmitted by food which has not been cooked or has been handled after cooking by a human who is a carrier of the virus. Inadequately cooked shellfish collected from sewage-contaminated waters are a common cause of viral food poisoning.

3. Chemical food poisoning The food is poisonous because it has been contaminated by chemicals during the growth, preparation, storage or cooking of the food. Most cases of chemical food poisoning are caused by carelessness in the home or an industrial establishment. Cleaning materials should be stored away from food and in such a way that they will not spill or leak from their containers. They must be clearly labelled and should never be decanted into food or drink containers. There are strict regulations for food producers and food manufacturers

10

governing the use of insecticidal sprays, pesticides, food additives and packaging materials. There have been a few outbreaks of zinc poisoning due to the use of galvanised equipment with acid foods. Chipped enamel vessels can cause antimony poisoning, particularly if used with acid foods.

4. *Vegetable food poisoning* Certain plants naturally contain substances which are poisonous to human beings, for example toadstools, hemlock, deadly nightshade, rhubarb leaves. The most common cause of vegetable food poisoning is the toadstool which can easily be mistaken for a mushroom. The consumption of raw or undercooked red kidney beans causes severe vomiting. The naturally occurring poison present in raw red kidney beans can be destroyed by boiling them for 10 minutes. Canned red kidney beans are quite safe to eat without further cooking.

BACTERIAL FOOD POISONING

How many bacteria must be present to cause illness?

Quite frequently we eat food which contains a few food poisoning bacteria but small numbers of most types of bacteria do not cause illness. Millions of bacteria must be present before a healthy adult will feel any harmful effects. A child under one year, an old person or a sick person would be affected by the presence of far fewer bacteria. Special care must therefore be taken when preparing food for people in these categories.

Food poisoning is occasionally fatal in this country. The deaths caused by food poisoning are usually in very young babies or in old or severely ill people.

Incubation period

This is the time that passes between the entry of the poisonous food into the body and the occurrence of the first symptoms. The length of the incubation period helps to decide which type of bacteria has caused the food poisoning. Some types of bacteria cause food poisoning with a relatively long incubation period (up to 2 days) and other types of bacteria cause food poisoning with a relatively short incubation period (2 hours). The length of the incubation period also depends on the number of bacteria present as well as the type of bacteria causing the food poisoning. If the food is very heavily contaminated with a certain type of bacteria, the incubation period will be shorter than if the food is contaminated with only half the number of the same type of bacteria.

Duration

The duration of the illness is the time between the appearance of the first symptoms of food poisoning and the clearing up of the last ones. When all the symptoms of food poisoning have gone, it does not necessarily mean that there are no harmful bacteria in the intestinal tract (see convalescent carriers p. 14).

THE BACTERIA WHICH CAUSE FOOD POISONING

The following bacteria frequently cause food poisoning:

> *Salmonella*
> *Staphylococcus aureus*
> *Clostridium perfringens*
> *Bacillus cereus*

All bacteria have two names:

The *generic name* which is written first and with a capital letter (equivalent to our surname), e.g. *Clostridium, Bacillus*. The *specific name* which is written with a small letter after the generic name (equivalent to our first names e.g. *perfringens, cereus.*

There are approximately 2000 species of the *Salmonella* genus (e.g. *Salmonella typhimurium, Salmonella enteritidis, Salmonella hadar, Salmonella newport*) but since most of them cause food poisoning it is usual to talk about *Salmonella* food poisoning without distinguishing which species is actually the cause. *Salmonella, Staphylococcus aureus, Clostridium perfringens* and *Bacillus cereus* are all common causes of food poisoning in the UK and many other countries. It is important to know how these particular bacteria normally gain access to food and what measures can be taken to avoid this or to prevent their multiplication.

Several other bacteria can cause food poisoning but do so far less frequently than those mentioned above (see Appendix).

SUMMARY

1. The symptoms of food poisoning are usually vomiting, diarrhoea and abdominal pains.

2. The four main types of food poisoning are:
   (a) Bacterial food poisoning — the most common.
   (b) Viral food poisoning.
   (c) Chemical food poisoning.
   (d) Vegetable food poisoning.

3. The incubation period and the duration of bacterial food poisoning give an indication of the type of bacteria which has caused the illness.

4. *Salmonella, Staphylococcus aureus, Clostridium perfringens* and *Bacillus cereus* frequently cause food poisoning in Britain and many other countries.

Chapter 4

Pathogenic Bacteria

HOW PATHOGENIC BACTERIA GAIN ACCESS TO THE KITCHEN

1. Raw meat

Animals and poultry frequently carry pathogenic bacteria in their intestines. When the animals are slaughtered and dressed, these bacteria may spread over the surface of the meat where they will grow and multiply rapidly unless the meat is refrigerated immediately and kept under refrigeration during transport and storage in the butcher's shop. If these storage rules are observed the bacteria on contaminated meat will remain dormant, but they will be able to grow and multiply again as soon as the meat is removed from refrigerated storage into normal room temperatures. However reputable the supplier, raw meat often carries small numbers of pathogenic bacteria. These will normally be killed in the cooking process, but care must be taken by the food handler not to let them have a chance to multiply and not to let them spread to foods which have already been cooked.

2. Food handlers

Pathogenic bacteria from food handlers can be spread into food, usually via the hands, during preparation and service. Everybody carries bacteria in their mouth, nose, intestine and on their skin and some of these bacteria will inevitably be transferred to food.

Carriers   A small percentage of the population are carriers of pathogenic bacteria and although they do not always have the symptoms of food poisoning, pathogenic bacteria are present in the intestinal tract and are therefore passed in their faeces. There are two types of carrier:

A *convalescent carrier* is someone who has recently recovered from food poisoning but is still harbouring pathogenic bacteria in the intestinal tract.

A *healthy carrier* is someone who has not suffered from food poisoning but is nevertheless carrying pathogenic bacteria in the intestinal tract.

Convalescent and healthy carriers run a high risk of contaminating their hands with food poisoning bacteria on visiting the toilet. A food handler who is excreting *Salmonella* bacteria is not allowed to work with food (see p. 119).

3. Animals and Insects

Flies, rats, mice, birds, other insects and animals including pets frequently carry pathogenic bacteria in their intestines and on their feet and fur and must therefore not be allowed to come into contact with food or equipment which will be used for food preparation.

4. Dust

Soil contains spores of some of the pathogenic bacteria. Raw vegetables must therefore always be cleaned thoroughly in a section of the kitchen used only for this purpose and then transferred to another section for further preparation.

All these carry food poisoning bacteria

CROSS-CONTAMINATION

Cross-contamination is the transfer of bacteria from a contaminated source to an uncontaminated food (usually freshly cooked food). If this food is suitable for bacterial growth and is left for some time in a warm room, the few bacteria which have been transferred to it will multiply to large numbers and when the food is eventually eaten it will cause food poisoning. If the original contaminated source was a raw food, it will not usually be a cause of food poisoning because the bacteria present are later destroyed by cooking.

Causes of cross-contamination   Bacteria can be transferred from a contaminated source to an uncontaminated food by:

(a) Using a chopping board, a working surface or other kitchen equipment for the preparation of raw and cooked foods without washing it thoroughly between each use.

(b) Using a knife or other utensil without washing it thoroughly between each use.

(c) The hands of a food handler which are not washed in between preparing different types of food, e.g. raw and cooked meat, or after touching any source of bacteria, e.g. the nose, mouth, hair, pets.

(d) Incorrect positioning of foods in a refrigerator. For example, raw meat must always be placed below cooked food so that blood (which often contains pathogenic bacteria) cannot drip on to the cooked food.

Examples of cross-contamination

1. *A mincer which has been used for raw meat and then for cooked corned beef.*
    A chef working in a busy kitchen is making liver pâté. He minces the raw liver and decides to leave cleaning the mincer until he has got the pâté into the oven.

    Before the first chef has finished the preparation of the pâté, a second chef uses the mincer for some corned beef which is to be used for a rissole. In this way, some bacteria from the liver are transferred to the corned beef.
    The rissoles are left in the kitchen for several hours before they are cooked. During this time the bacteria increase to a sufficient number to cause food poisoning. As all the ingredients in the rissoles have already

been cooked, they are only lightly browned before serving and the temperature reached in the centre of the rissoles during cooking is not sufficiently high to kill all the bacteria.

How food poisoning could have been prevented: By thoroughly washing the mincer immediately after use.

2. *A knife which has been used for cutting raw meat and not washed thoroughly before it is used for slicing cooked meat.*

A chef is preparing sandwiches for a children's picnic. He has just finished cutting up raw meat for a casserole and as he is in a hurry he gives his knife a quick wipe on his overall and continues to use it to slice some ham.

A smear of blood from the raw meat is left on the knife and when the cooked ham is sliced with the same knife a few pathogenic bacteria are transferred to it. The ham is then used to make sandwiches.

It is a warm day and before the sandwiches are eaten the bacteria increase to sufficient numbers to cause food poisoning.

How food poisoning could have been prevented: By using a different knife to cut the ham or by thoroughly washing the knife after using it for the raw meat and before using it for the cooked meat.

3. *A chef develops a heavy cold but does not report it to his employer and continues to work as usual on the preparation of desserts.*

While piping cream on to a trifle the chef sneezes. He naturally turns away from the food and sneezes into his handkerchief but he does not wash his hands before continuing with his work. A few bacteria from the handkerchief are transferred to his hands and from there to the cream on the trifle. The trifle is put on the sweet trolley and most of it is eaten fairly quickly but two portions remain for several hours in the warm dining room. Those who ate the trifle at the beginning of the evening did not develop food poisoning but by the time the final two portions were eaten the bacteria had increased to a sufficient number to cause illness.

How food poisoning could have been prevented: By washing his hands after touching the handkerchief. It is preferable to use disposable paper handkerchiefs which are destroyed after one use.

4. *Uncooked steak is placed on the top shelf of the refrigerator and uncovered roast chicken on the bottom shelf.*

A drop of blood from the uncooked steak drips on to the uncovered roast chicken stored below it.

A few pathogenic bacteria in the drop of blood are transferred to the chicken. They do not multiply in the refrigerator but remain dormant.

The chicken is served at a buffet on a warm afternoon. It is on display for three hours before it is eaten and during this time the bacteria increase to sufficient numbers to cause food poisoning.

How food poisoning could have been prevented: By using different refrigerators for storing raw and cooked meat or by placing the uncooked steak at the bottom of the refrigerator and the cooked chicken at the top.

COLOUR CODING OF EQUIPMENT

In order to avoid cross-contamination, equipment such as chopping boards and knives should be used for the preparation of only one type of food. A colour coding system (in which a small coloured tag is fixed to the equipment) is a way of identifying which equipment should be used for which type of food.

Colour code	Equipment to be used only for:
Red	Raw meat and poultry
Green	Fruits and vegetables
Blue	Raw fish
Brown	Cooked meats
White	Dairy products

SUMMARY

1. The main sources of pathogenic bacteria in the kitchen are raw meat, food handlers, animals, insects and dust.

2. Cross-contamination is the transfer of bacteria from a contaminated source to uncontaminated food.

3. Colour coding of equipment helps to prevent cross-contamination.

Chapter 5

Salmonella

Salmonella is a short, thin, rod-shaped bacterium.

Salmonella × 6400

More outbreaks of food poisoning in the UK are caused by *Salmonella* than by any other bacteria.

People can be severely ill with *Salmonella* food poisoning and there are between twenty and fifty fatal cases each year, usually in elderly, very young or sick people.

TYPE OF FOOD POISONING

Salmonella causes infective food poisoning.

Large numbers of living bacteria must be present in the food when it is eaten. Some of them will be destroyed by the acid in the stomach but some will be protected by food and pass through to the small intestine where the near neutral conditions allow them to multiply. As they increase in numbers, some of the cells die and release a poisonous substance which causes fever, diarrhoea and vomiting. Since it takes some time for the bacteria to increase in numbers to a level which causes symptoms, the incubation period is relatively long.

Incubation period	12–36 hours
Duration of illness	1–8 days
Symptoms	Fever, headache, abdominal pains, diarrhoea and vomiting

NATURAL ORIGIN OF *SALMONELLA*

1. *Salmonella* is commonly found in animal fodder and is therefore found in the intestines of many farm animals, particularly poultry.

2. Mice, rats, domestic pets, flies and birds also often carry *Salmonella* in their intestines and on their fur and feet.

MEANS OF ACCESS TO FOOD

1. Brought into the kitchen on or in foods of animal origin, e.g. poultry, meat, unpasteurised milk, dried egg powder.

   Salmonella is normally present only on the surface of raw meat but is often present in the central cavity of poultry or in the centre of minced meat products such as sausages and hamburgers. These foods may cause poisoning if they are inadequately cooked or they may contaminate other foods which have already been cooked.

   Unpasteurised milk is sometimes contaminated with *Salmonella*. Pasteurisation destroys *Salmonella*.

   Duck eggs frequently harbour *Salmonella* and it has recently been found that some hen eggs do but it is thought to be only a small proportion. The shell of both types may be contaminated with *Salmonella*.

2. Insects, birds, vermin and domestic pets can spread *Salmonella* into food if they are allowed to be present in the kitchen.

3. People working in the kitchen are sometimes, unknown to them, carrying *Salmonella* in their intestines and may contaminate food if they don't wash their hands after a visit to the toilet.

DESTRUCTION

Salmonella is readily killed by heat. It does not form a spore.

FOODS USUALLY INVOLVED

Foods causing this type of food poisoning have either been cooked inadequately or have been contaminated after cooking, e.g. poultry which has not been properly defrosted, cold meats which have been cross-contaminated.

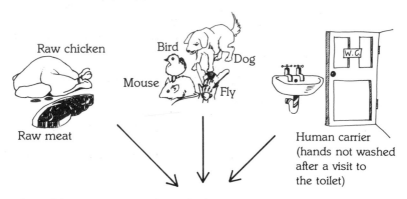

Raw chicken

Raw meat

Bird

Dog

Mouse

Fly

Human carrier
(hands not washed
after a visit to
the toilet)

Any of these may contaminate the foods below with *Salmonella*

These foods are not cooked again

They are kept warm for several hours

FOOD POISONING

PREVENTIVE MEASURES

1. Thaw frozen food completely before cooking. Allow 24 hours to thaw a 3 lb (1.5 kg) chicken in the refrigerator. A large turkey would take too long to thaw in a refrigerator and should be thawed in a chiller or a cool area of the kitchen.

2. Cook food thoroughly making sure the temperature at the centre of the food is high enough to kill bacteria.

3. Use different surfaces and equipment e.g. chopping boards, knives, etc. for preparing raw food and cooked food.

4. Clean all equipment thoroughly after each use.

5. Store raw and cooked foods (particularly meat) separately.

6. Wash hands after handling raw meat, poultry and eggs.

7. Keep food as cold as possible to prevent multiplication of Salmonella.

A TYPICAL CHAIN OF EVENTS LEADING TO FOOD POISONING BY SALMONELLA

Roast chicken is a favourite on the menu at a restaurant where many people have their midday meal. Normally the chickens are taken from the deep freeze the previous evening and left to defrost in the refrigerator overnight.

One evening the chef forgot to remove the chickens from the deep freeze so he arrived at work early the next morning and put them in a sink of hot water for two hours. He then ran some hot water inside the chicken carcasses and managed to melt some of the ice. He hastily stuffed the chickens and put them into the oven to cook for lunchtime thinking that the rest of the ice would melt in the heat of the oven.

After the normal cooking time he was relieved to find that the flesh appeared to be perfectly cooked and so he served it at lunchtime as usual with a portion of stuffing.

The following day several people in the area have to go to their doctors with severe headaches, abdominal pains, diarrhoea and vomiting. They are questioned about where they had eaten their meals during the last 36 hours and an outbreak of Salmonella food poisoning is traced to the restaurant where the chickens were served.

The chickens are almost defrosted, so they are stuffed and put in the oven to cook

Lunch is served

12.30 p.m.

10.30 a.m.

8 a.m.

During the day, all those who had eaten the chicken the day before became ill

6 a.m.

Chef arrives early to remove the chickens from the deep-freeze

DAY 1

After a restless night, the first victim wakes up feeling sick, and with abdominal pains

DAY 2

Fault

Frozen meat, particularly poultry, must be thawed completely before commencing cooking. If ice is present in the centre of the chicken, a great deal of heat is used to melt it. It will take far longer for the internal temperature to equal the external temperature than it would if the chicken were completely defrosted. Even if the chicken is cooked for the recommended time, the temperature in the centre of the bird at the end of the cooking time is not sufficiently high to kill *Salmonella* but is probably an optimum temperature for its multiplication. It is advisable to cook stuffing separately and not in the bird, where it will slow down heat penetration.

Chapter 6

Staphylococcus aureus

Staphylococcus aureus is a round bacterium.

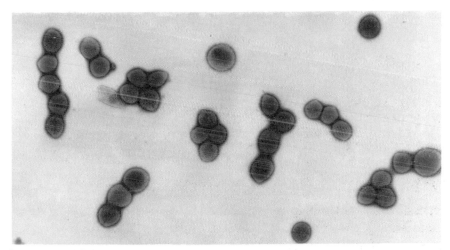

S. aureus × 6400

The symptoms of food poisoning caused by *Staphylococcus aureus* are severe for a short period of time but the illness is rarely fatal.

TYPE OF FOOD POISONING

Staphylococcus aureus causes toxic food poisoning. Whilst growing and multiplying in food stored at a warm temperature, it produces a toxin (a poisonous substance). When the food is swallowed the toxin irritates the stomach lining causing vomiting. The incubation period is therefore relatively short and the main symptom is vomiting.

Incubation period   1–7 hours

Duration of illness   6–24 hours

Symptoms   Vomiting, sometimes abdominal pains and diarrhoea

NATURAL ORIGIN OF *STAPHYLOCOCCUS AUREUS*

Staphylococcus aureus is frequently present in the human nose and throat and on the skin of healthy people. It is known as a commensal because it is completely harmless when present in these areas. It is found also in large numbers in boils, styes and septic cuts.

Staphylococcus aureus is sometimes present in unpasteurised milk.

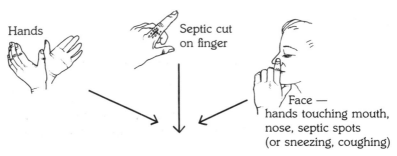

Hands

Septic cut on finger

Face — hands touching mouth, nose, septic spots (or sneezing, coughing)

Any of these may contaminate the foods below with *Staphylococcus aureus*

These foods are lightly cooked or not cooked at all

They are kept warm for several hours

FOOD POISONING

MEANS OF ACCESS TO FOOD

1. People working in the kitchen who sneeze or cough over food or who have septic cuts, boils, styes, etc. and do not cover them with an adequate waterproof dressing.

2. Unpasteurised milk and products made from unpasteurised milk which are not cooked or only lightly cooked.

DESTRUCTION

Staphylococcus aureus does not form a spore and is therefore readily killed by heat (1–2 minutes in boiling water) BUT the toxin which it produces in food is more resistant to heat than the bacterial cell and can withstand up to 30 minutes in boiling water. It is therefore possible for lightly cooked food to contain active toxin but no live bacteria. This food will still cause food poisoning.

FOODS USUALLY INVOLVED

Foods causing Staphylococcus aureus food poisoning are usually those which have been contaminated by the food handler after they have been cooked and are then eaten cold or after a mild reheating process, e.g. sliced cold meats, cream dishes, custards and other milk products and stuffed rolled joints which have not been cooked through to the centre. Staphylococcus is able to grow in higher concentrations of salt than the other food poisoning bacteria and therefore outbreaks involving salty foods, e.g. ham, are often traced to Staphylococcus.

PREVENTIVE MEASURES

1. Maintain a high standard of personal hygiene.

2. Handle food as little as possible. Always use serving tongs for food which will not be heated again.

3. Keep food as cold as possible to prevent the multiplication of Staphylococcus aureus.

A TYPICAL CHAIN OF EVENTS LEADING TO
FOOD POISONING BY *STAPHYLOCOCCUS AUREUS*

At a school canteen, custard is served most days with the pudding. As it is fairly easy to prepare, a new member of staff was allocated this task. He starts work at 8.00 a.m. and on one particular morning as there is no other urgent work, he starts by preparing the custard. At 8.30 a.m. he moves on to another task and leaves the custard to cool but suddenly wonders if he remembered to add the sugar. He tastes it with a spoon and thinks it seems sweet enough but just checks it again using the same spoon without washing it. He is then quite satisfied that the sugar has been added. The custard is left in the kitchen for the rest of the morning and at 12.15 p.m. it is warmed up and served for lunch at 12.30 p.m.

That afternoon several children start to feel sick and have acute stomach pains. By 5.30 p.m. that evening many of the children who had eaten the custard are ill and an outbreak of food poisoning caused by *Staphylococcus aureus* is confirmed.

Custard is served

Custard is tasted for sweetness

12.30 p.m.

Children start to feel ill

9 a.m.
8.30 a.m.
8 a.m.
3 p.m.

Custard is left to cool

5.30 p.m.

Custard is prepared

Many of the children who ate the custard are sick

Fault

A spoon which has been put into the mouth must never be returned to food without first washing it. *Staphylococcus aureus* may be transferred from the mouth to food via the spoon. If the food is left for some time at a warm temperature the bacteria will grow, multiply and produce toxins. If the food is only lightly reheated the toxins will not be destroyed.

Chapter 7

Clostridium perfringens

Clostridium perfringens is a rod-shaped bacterium. It can form a spore when conditions are unfavourable for growth and is also an anaerobe so grows best in the absence of oxygen.

C. perfringens × 6400

Clostridium perfringens food poisoning is rarely fatal.

TYPE OF FOOD POISONING

Clostridium perfringens does not produce toxin when it is multiplying in food stored at a warm temperature, but when that food is eaten the bacteria form spores and at the same time a toxin, which irritates the intestinal wall causing diarrhoea. This is not exactly the same as toxic food poisoning or infective food poisoning but has some characteristics of both. The incubation period is longer than with toxic food poisoning as caused by *Staphylococcus aureus* and shorter than infective food poisoning as caused by *Salmonella*.

Incubation period	8–22 hours
Duration of illness	12–24 hours
Symptoms	Abdominal pains and diarrhoea. The patient rarely vomits.

NATURAL ORIGIN OF *CLOSTRIDIUM PERFRINGENS*

1. *C. perfringens* is frequently present in human and animal intestines.

2. Flies and bluebottles are usually heavily infected with *C. perfringens*.

3. Spores of *C. perfringens* are found in soil.

Any of these may contaminate the foods below with *C. perfringens*

C. perfringens is not destroyed by cooking

Food kept at a warm temperature for several hours

FOOD POISONING

MEANS OF ACCESS TO FOOD

1. Brought into the kitchen on raw meat. The meat itself may cause food poisoning since *C. perfringens* can survive cooking processes by forming a spore. Bacteria from the raw meat may also be transferred to cooked foods in careless preparation.

2. Vegetables coated with soil, or dust from sacks or packing cases may contaminate foods with *C. perfringens* if the soil or dust settles on food.

3. People working in the kitchen may be carrying *C. perfringens* in their intestines and may spread the bacteria into food if their hands are not washed after a visit to the toilet.

DESTRUCTION

The spores of *C. perfringens* are not destroyed by normal cooking methods. They can withstand boiling, steaming, stewing or braising for up to 4 hours. The spores do not multiply but if the food is cooled slowly and kept warm for some time before serving, the spores germinate producing vegetative bacteria which multiply rapidly.

FOODS USUALLY INVOLVED

As it does not grow readily in the presence of oxygen, *C. perfringens* is most frequently found reproducing rapidly at the bottom of a lukewarm meat casserole or stock pot or at the centre of large food masses where there is little air (oxygen), e.g. meat pies, minced meat dishes. Reheated meat dishes are also frequently a cause of *C. perfringens* food poisoning since the spore it forms will survive each reheating process.

Most outbreaks involve a large number of people because *C. perfringens* is more commonly found in foods that have been prepared in bulk.

PREVENTIVE MEASURES

1. Use separate preparation areas for raw food (especially meat and vegetables) and cooked food.

2. Cool cooked foods rapidly and refrigerate promptly. To do this it may be necessary to break up large volumes of meat and cool and store it in separate smaller containers. Large joints of meat should be removed from the cooking liquor immediately after cooking to speed up cooling.

3. Use different surfaces and equipment e.g. chopping boards, knives, etc. for preparing raw food and cooked food.

4. Clean all equipment thoroughly after each use.

5. Store raw foods (particularly meat and unwashed vegetables) away from cooked food.

6. Wash hands after handling raw meat and unwashed vegetables.

7. If reheating of food is necessary, it must be reheated rapidly and thoroughly and then served quickly. Never reheat meat products more than once.

A TYPICAL CHAIN OF EVENTS LEADING TO FOOD POISONING BY *CLOSTRIDIUM PERFRINGENS*

The staff in a works canteen are responsible for preparing a main meal for all the people at the factory. There are two shifts. The early shift eats lunch at 11.00 a.m. The late shift eats at 2.00 p.m.

One day, one of the dishes on the menu is beef casserole. The chef preparing the casserole gathers together the ingredients (beef, onions, carrots and swedes) and takes them to the working surface where he usually does his preparation. He cuts the beef and puts it on one side and then scrapes the vegetables, chops them and puts everything together in the casserole which is then cooked in time for the first shift. It is taken from the oven a few minutes before 11.00 a.m. and served piping hot to the people on the first shift. However, not all of it is used so rather than see it wasted the staff decide to leave it in the warming cabinet to keep it warm for the second shift. The temperature in the warming cabinet is 45 °C.

That night some of the people from the factory start to feel ill with severe abdominal pains and diarrhoea. An outbreak of food poisoning caused by *C. perfringens* is confirmed and traced to the beef casserole although it is only the people on the second shift who are ill and none of those from the first shift are affected.

People on the first shift have lunch. Some of them choose beef casserole

Some of the people from the factory wake up with abdominal pains and diarrhoea

People on the second shift have lunch. Some of them choose beef casserole

11 a.m.

2 p.m.

1 a.m.

8 a.m.

Chef prepares the beef casserole and puts it in the oven to cook

During the night many of those from the second shift who ate beef casserole are ill

DAY 1

DAY 2

Faults

1. Separate working areas, equipment and utensils should be used for preparing raw meat and vegetables.

2. Foods which are suitable for bacterial growth should never be kept warm. If they are not served immediately they must be kept hot, at a temperature above 63 °C or cold, at a temperature below 8 °C. In this case the casserole was kept warm for three hours in between servings. *C. perfringens* from either the raw meat or from soil on the vegetables had survived the cooking process by forming spores which were able to germinate, grow and multiply rapidly when the casserole was kept at a temperature of 45 °C.

Chapter 8

Bacillus cereus

Bacillus cereus is a rod–shaped bacterium. It can form a spore when conditions are unfavourable for growth. It is an aerobe and therefore requires oxygen for growth.

B. cereus × 6400

The onset of symptoms of *Bacillus cereus* food poisoning can be very sudden but it is usually over fairly quickly. It is most unlikely to be fatal.

TYPE OF FOOD POISONING

Bacillus cereus usually causes toxic food poisoning. Whilst *B. cereus* is growing and multiplying in food stored at a warm temperature, it produces a toxin. When the food is swallowed the toxin irritates the stomach lining causing vomiting.

Incubation period	1–5 hours
Duration	6–24 hours
Symptoms	Vomiting, abdominal pains, occasionally diarrhoea

There is a second type of *B. cereus* food poisoning which is rare in the United Kingdom. Toxins are produced in the intestine but not in the food before it is eaten. The incubation period is longer and the main symptom is diarrhoea.

NATURAL ORIGIN OF *BACILLUS CEREUS*

Bacillus cereus is found in the soil and in dust.

MEANS OF ACCESS TO FOOD

The spores of *B. cereus* are brought into the kitchen on cereals, particularly rice. Cornflour and spices are also often contaminated.

DESTRUCTION

The spores of *B. cereus* are not easily destroyed by heat and will survive most cooking processes. They do not multiply but if the food is cooled slowly or kept warm for some time before serving, they will germinate producing vegetative bacteria which multiply rapidly at these temperatures and produce a very heat-resistant toxin. If the food is subsequently reheated quickly, the heat is unlikely to be sufficient to destroy the toxin.

FOODS USUALLY INVOLVED

Reheated rice is almost always the cause of *B. cereus* food poisoning.

PREVENTIVE MEASURES

1. Cool cooked food rapidly and refrigerate promptly.
2. If reheating of the food is necessary, it must be reheated rapidly and thoroughly and then served quickly. Never reheat rice more than once.

A TYPICAL CHAIN OF EVENTS LEADING TO FOOD POISONING BY *B. CEREUS*

A housewife has invited twelve friends for a buffet supper party after a visit to the theatre. She has planned to cook a curry and serve it with plain boiled rice. She knows she will not have time to prepare the curry on the evening of the party so she prepares it on the previous evening and after cooking it she cools it quickly and puts it in the refrigerator to store overnight. She also cooks the rice the night before but as there is no room in the refrigerator she covers it and leaves it on the working surface in the kitchen thinking that rice is a 'safe' food anyway.

The next evening, just before the guests arrive, she reheats the curry thoroughly and then warms the rice through over a pan of boiling water and serves both to the guests.

Even before the party is over, several of the guests suddenly start to feel very sick and some of the others are ill during the night. An outbreak of food poisoning due to *B. cereus* is traced to the rice.

The rice is cooked and left to cool

8 p.m.

7 p.m.

The curry is cooked, cooled and refrigerated promptly

DAY 1

The curry and rice are served to the guests

10.30 p.m.

10 p.m.

1 a.m.

Some of the guests start to feel ill

The curry and rice are reheated

DAY 2 — DAY 3

Fault

Bacteria which had survived the first cooking of the rice by forming spores had germinated into vegetative bacteria, multiplied and produced toxin during long slow cooling overnight. The rice was not reheated sufficiently to destroy the toxin in it.

THE BACTERIA WHICH COMMONLY CAUSE FOOD POISONING

	Salmonella	*Staphylococcus*	*C. perfringens*	*B. cereus*
Incuba-tion period	12–36 hours	1–7 hours	8–22 hours	1–5 hours
Duration of illness	1–8 days	6–24 hours	12–24 hours	6–24 hours
Means of access to the kitchen	Poultry and other raw meat. Animals. Human carriers	Mainly through humans, from the nose, mouth, infected wounds and sores	Raw meat. Unwashed vegetables. Human carriers	Cereals especially rice
Foods usually involved	Meat and meat products	Almost any food which has been handled and not cooked or only lightly cooked afterwards, e.g. sliced cold meats, cream and milk products	Meat dishes, e.g. stews, pies, gravy, meat stock. Unwashed vegetables.	Rice
Destruc-tion	Vegetative bacteria readily destroyed by heat. Does not form spores. Does not produce a toxin	Vegetative bacteria readily destroyed by heat. Does not form spores. Toxin destroyed by boiling for 30 mins	Forms spores which can survive several hours in boiling water. Therefore not normally destroyed in cooking processes	Forms spores which can survive several hours in boiling water, therefore not normally destroyed in cooking processes

THE HUMAN DIGESTIVE SYSTEM

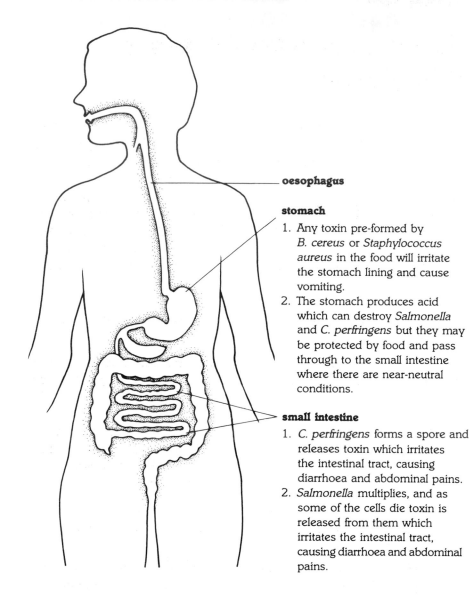

oesophagus

stomach

1. Any toxin pre-formed by *B. cereus* or *Staphylococcus aureus* in the food will irritate the stomach lining and cause vomiting.
2. The stomach produces acid which can destroy *Salmonella* and *C. perfringens* but they may be protected by food and pass through to the small intestine where there are near-neutral conditions.

small intestine

1. *C. perfringens* forms a spore and releases toxin which irritates the intestinal tract, causing diarrhoea and abdominal pains.
2. *Salmonella* multiplies, and as some of the cells die toxin is released from them which irritates the intestinal tract, causing diarrhoea and abdominal pains.

Chapter 9

Bacterial Food-Borne Diseases

There are many food-borne diseases, several of which are far more serious than the food poisoning caused by *Salmonella, Staphylococcus aureus, Clostridium perfringens* and *Bacillus cereus*. Some are caused by bacteria. Others are caused by viruses, protozoa or parasitic worms (see Appendix).

Bacterial food-borne diseases differ from bacterial food poisoning in that illness is caused by the ingestion of only small numbers of bacteria whereas large numbers of bacteria, or the toxin produced by them, must be ingested to cause the acute vomiting and diarrhoea known as food poisoning.

Bacterial food-borne diseases	Bacterial food poisoning
e.g. *Campylobacter* infection, dysentery, typhoid, paratyphoid, cholera,	Caused by *Salmonella, Staphylococcus aureus, C. perfringens, B. cereus*
1. Relatively small numbers of the bacteria can cause illness.	1. Large numbers of the bacteria or toxin produced by them must be ingested before any ill effects are felt.
2. Contaminated drinking water frequently transmits these diseases.	2. Contaminated drinking water does not cause food poisoning.
3. The incubation period is fairly long: 1–25 days.	3. The incubation period is relatively short: 2–36 hours.

Food-borne diseases are frequently transmitted by contaminated drinking water, by food which has been washed in it, by shellfish or watercress gathered from it or by dehydrated food which has been rehydrated with it. After a natural disaster such as an earthquake or flooding, the drinking water sometimes becomes contaminated with sewage causing large outbreaks of these diseases.

Campylobacter infection

Bacteria called *Campylobacter jejuni* and *Campylobacter coli* are the commonest cause of diarrhoea in the UK.

Reported cases of illness attributed to *Campylobacter*					
1989	*1990*	*1991*	*1992*	*1993*	*1994*
32 526	34 552	32 636	38 552	39 385	44 317

Source: Public Health Laboratory Service Communicable Disease Surveillance Centre

Incubation period 3–5 days

Symptoms Flu-like symptoms for the first 24 hours, followed by stomach cramps and severe diarrhoea which usually lasts from 1–10 days.

Cause of the disease There is still much to be learnt about the cause of this disease. Many farm animals (cows, sheep and chickens) and domestic pets (cats, dogs) carry *Campylobacter* without showing any symptoms of illness. Some human infections are probably as a result of direct contact with these animals but most of the outbreaks have been traced to the consumption of undercooked chicken, unpasteurised milk and pasteurised milk drunk from bottles which have been pecked by birds on the doorstep. Non-mains water in the UK and water in developing countries is also known to transmit *Campylobacter* infection. Bacteria from the genus *Campylobacter* are not heat resistant.

Dysentery

There are two types of dysentery:

Bacillary dysentery is caused by several species of the genus *Shigella*. Outbreaks involving large numbers occur regularly in the UK.

Incubation period 1–7 days

Symptoms Severe diarrhoea and fever. Sometimes vomiting.

Natural origin of the bacteria *Shigella* is a parasite of humans only and therefore if an outbreak occurs there must be a human carrier involved at some stage.

Causes of the disease

1. Personal contact. Bacillary dysentery can spread quickly in schools and institutions especially if personal hygiene standards are low (faecal-oral transmission).

2. Food handlers who are carriers of *Shigella* and have contaminated food by failing to wash their hands after a visit to the toilet.

Amoebic dysentery   This disease is rare in Europe. It is caused by a protozoan (see p. 126).

Typhoid fever

Typhoid fever is caused by *Salmonella typhi*. It is a more severe form of illness than the food poisoning caused by the majority of species of the *Salmonella* genus. Typhoid fever is rare in the United Kingdom but occasionally people suffer on returning from a trip abroad. After the illness some people become convalescent carriers for the rest of their lives.

Incubation period	7–21 days
Symptoms	Prolonged fever with rose-coloured spots on the body. Severe diarrhoea usually commences in the second or third week of the fever. Typhoid fever is fatal in 2–10 per cent of all cases.

Natural origin of the bacteria   *Salmonella typhi* is a parasite of humans only, unlike most other *Salmonellae* which are found in a wide variety of animals.

Causes of the disease

1. Food handlers who are carriers of *Salmonella typhi* and have contaminated food by failing to wash their hands after a visit to the toilet. People who are confirmed carriers of *Salmonella typhi* are not allowed to work in the food industry.

2. Drinking water that has been contaminated by sewage.

3. In a few instances, shellfish and watercress gathered from sewage-contaminated water have caused typhoid. Laws governing the gathering and cleansing of shellfish have more or less eliminated them as a cause of typhoid fever. Watercress should always be thoroughly washed.

Paratyphoid fever

Paratyphoid fever is caused by *Salmonella paratyphi.*

Incubation period   1–10 days

Symptoms   Fever, diarrhoea. Paratyphoid fever is similar to
                             typhoid fever but the symptoms are generally
                             less severe.

Natural origin of the bacteria   Human carriers.

Causes of the disease

1. Food handlers who are carriers of *Salmonella paratyphi.*

2. Drinking water that has been contaminated by sewage.

3. Food gathered from contaminated water.

Cholera

Cholera is a severe illness caused by a bacterium called *Vibrio cholerae.*
It usually occurs as a result of eating food washed in sewage-
contaminated water or by drinking the water itself. The symptoms are
very severe diarrhoea and vomiting resulting in dehydration of the
patient. The illness is often fatal and all visitors to countries where
cholera is common should be vaccinated against it. Re-vaccination is
required every six months.

SUMMARY

1. A food-borne disease caused by *Campylobacter* is the most
    common cause of diarrhoea in the UK.

2. Outbreaks of bacillary dysentery involving large numbers of people
    occur regularly in the UK.

3. Typhoid, paratyphoid and cholera are food-borne diseases that are
    rare in the UK.

Chapter 10

Personal Hygiene and Kitchen Hygiene

There are two aspects to the prevention of food poisoning.

1. A food handler must as far as possible prevent bacteria from entering food by maintaining a high standard of personal hygiene and by being aware of all possible sources of contamination in the kitchen.

2. A food handler must discourage the multiplication of any bacteria which may be present so that the numbers never become sufficiently large to cause an outbreak of food poisoning. This can be done by cooking and storing foods correctly (see chapter 11).

HAND WASHING

Food poisoning bacteria carried on the hands and transferred into food during its preparation are one of the most common causes of food contamination.

Before washing

After washing

Nutrient agar plates showing bacteria originating from unwashed and washed hands

In all catering establishments, by law, there must be sufficient wash basins in places where the food handlers can reach them quickly and easily from where they are working. Wash basins and nail brushes must also be provided near the toilets. Wash hand-basins should not be used for food washing and hands should not be washed in sinks used for the preparation of food or for washing-up.

Before commencing food preparation, hands and forearms should always be washed with hot water and soap and not just rinsed under the tap. A liquid soap dispenser is more hygienic than a soap tablet which is used by everybody. Some soaps are called bactericidal soaps because they contain a disinfectant which helps to reduce the number of bacteria on the hands.

Nails should always be kept short and should be scrubbed whenever the hands are washed because bacteria will collect under them. Nail varnish should not be worn when preparing foods as it easily chips and could fall into food.

Towels rapidly become contaminated with bacteria and an individual method of hand drying is essential. This can either be paper towels together with a foot operated disposal bin, a linen roller towel or a hot-air drier.

Hygienic methods of hand drying

After thorough drying, hand cream with added disinfectant should be used to keep the skin in good condition. Cracks and grooves in the skin surface or round the nails or knuckles usually harbour *Staphylococci* bacteria which are not easily removed when the hands are washed.

Hands must always be washed before handling food but even so unnecessary handling of food should be avoided. Where possible clean serving tongs should be used, especially for foods which are to be eaten without further cooking, e.g. cream cakes, cooked meats.

It is very important to wash the hands after:	**Reason**
1. Visiting the toilet.	Bacteria in the faeces can get through toilet paper on to the hands and so on to food.

2. Blowing the nose.	Many people harbour *Staphylococci* bacteria in their noses. Some of these bacteria will be transferred to the hands when a handkerchief is handled. It is preferable to use disposable handkerchiefs which are destroyed after *one* use.

3. Handling raw meat, poultry or vegetables.

The transfer of bacteria from raw meat to cooked dishes (cross-contamination) is a frequent cause of food poisoning. Many raw meat samples have food poisoning bacteria (usually *Cl. perfringens* or *Salmonella*) on the surface. Soil usually contains spores of *Cl. perfringens*.

Nutrient agar plate showing presence of bacteria on the hand after handling raw meat

Nutrient agar plate showing presence of bacteria on the hand after washing vegetables coated with soil

4. Breaking eggs.

Salmonella is often present on eggshells.

5. After handling refuse or contaminated food.

A great number of all types of bacteria will be present in refuse and waste food.

Under no circumstances should food handlers:

1. Smoke in the kitchen.

Reason

It is forbidden by law because bacteria can be transferred from the mouth and lips to the hands. Also, ash may drop into the food.

2. Sneeze or cough over food.

Droplets of moisture expelled during coughing and sneezing carry large numbers of *Staphylococci* bacteria to the food or working surfaces.

Nutrient agar plate showing bacterial growth produced by a sneeze

3. Comb their hair in the kitchen.

Staphylococci bacteria grow well on the scalp and will be transferred to the hands. Loose hairs and dandruff could fall on nearby food. Hair must be washed regularly and covered with a net or hat whilst working in the kitchen.

4. Dip their fingers into food to taste it, lick a spoon and return it to the food without washing it, or lick their fingers to separate sheets of wrapping paper.

Bacteria will be transferred from the mouth to the hands, spoon or paper and so to food.

5. Wear any jewellery other than plain wedding rings whilst working in the kitchen.

The skin under jewellery tends to harbour a large number of bacteria especially if the jewellery is not removed in washing. There is always a risk that earrings, tie pins, cufflinks, dress rings, etc. could fall off and become mixed with the food.

It is the duty of every food handler to:

Reason

1. Cover cuts and sores with a coloured waterproof dressing which must be changed regularly. Anyone with a septic cut or a boil, whitlow or stye should stop working with food until it is completely healed.

Any cut or sore is likely to be harbouring *Staphylococci* bacteria. If a coloured dressing accidentally falls off it will be seen before the food is used. If this does happen all the food in the same container must be discarded. It is not satisfactory merely to remove the dressing from the food. Septic cuts, boils, styes, and whitlows contain millions of *Staphylococci* bacteria.

2. Report any illness, however mild, to his supervisor who will decide whether he is fit to work. This applies particularly to diarrhoea and vomiting, throat and skin infections.

Diarrhoea and vomiting are symptoms of food poisoning and even if the condition has cleared up, the employee may still be a convalescent carrier. *Staphylococci* bacteria are normally present in throat and skin infections.

Health Education
Council poster

52

3. Wear clean overalls, aprons and headgear. Keep sleeves rolled up or securely fastened at the wrists so that cuffs cannot dip into food.

Outdoor clothing is frequently contaminated with *Staphylococci* particularly if it has been worn in congested areas such as on public transport. Clothing lockers should be situated outside the kitchen, making it possible to change into clean, protective clothing before handling food.

4. Use clean utensils for food preparation. Separate work surfaces and chopping boards should be set aside for the preparation of raw meat and must not be used for the preparation of foods which will be eaten without further cooking.

The transfer of bacteria from raw food to cooked food via kitchen utensils or work surfaces is frequently a cause of food poisoning.

5. Pick up knives and forks by their handles, glasses by the stems and plates by the edges.

Bacteria on the hands can be passed to cutlery and crockery and from these articles back to food.

6. Discard any chipped plates, glasses and damaged utensils.

Even an efficient washing-up process may fail to remove bacteria from cracks.

7. Cover food on display.

Flies will be attracted to uncovered food and bacteria in dust particles will settle on the food if it is left uncovered.

8. Keep pets out of the kitchen.

All animals carry bacteria on their feet and in their fur and these can easily spread into food if the animals are allowed to wander freely in the kitchen.

9. Keep pet food away from human food, using separate utensils for its preparation.

Pet food (except canned pet food) is usually heavily contaminated with bacteria.

FOREIGN BODIES IN FOOD

It is the duty of a food handler and anyone who services equipment to be used for food preparation to ensure that foreign bodies do not find their way into food. The following list gives examples of foreign bodies that have been found in food.

Foreign body	Prevention
1. Bolts, nuts, wire	Take great care with small parts of equipment during cleaning and maintenance work.
2. Cardboard, string, staples, paper, polythene, wood splinters	Do not unpack goods near open food.
3. Earrings, false finger nails, buttons, pen-tops	Wear only plain wedding rings when preparing food.
4. Sweet papers and cigarette ends	Do not smoke or eat whilst preparing food.
5. Glass	Discard any food from a broken or chipped container. Ensure that all glass is cleaned away after a breakage.
6. Cat, dog and animal hairs, feathers	Do not allow animals into an industrial kitchen and ensure it is kept free of pests.

SUMMARY

Maintaining a high standard of personal cleanliness and reporting all illnesses will reduce the risk of causing food poisoning.

Chapter 11

The Control of Bacterial Growth

If the precautions listed in Chapter 10 are observed during food preparation there should be very few harmful bacteria added to the food and certainly not a sufficiently large number to cause food poisoning. However, the following precautions must be taken so that if some pathogenic bacteria were originally present in the food or have inadvertently entered during preparation, they will be prevented from multiplying.

1. Thaw all frozen meat completely before cooking

It is essential that all frozen meats (particularly poultry) should be thawed completely before commencing cooking. If ice is present in the centre of meat it will take far longer for the internal temperature to reach that of the external temperature than in completely defrosted meat. *Salmonella* food poisoning has frequently been caused because chickens have not been thoroughly defrosted. Although they have been cooked for the recommended time, a great deal of heat is used to melt the remaining ice and the temperature reached in the centre of the bird is not sufficiently high to kill *Salmonella* but is an optimum temperature for its multiplication.

2. Cook food thoroughly

Food is a poor conductor of heat and it takes a long time before the temperature in the centre reaches the same temperature as at the surface. For this reason it is safer to reduce the size of rolled joints and minced meats to a maximum of 3 kg (6.6 lb) before cooking them.

Meat and meat products containing raw meat should never be partly cooked one day and the cooking process finished the next day. If the food is only partly cooked it is likely that bacteria will still be alive, and even if it is stored in a refrigerator there will be time for bacteria to multiply during the cooling down process and the second heating process. Just as the centre of joints of meat and meat products only slowly reaches the external temperature when heated up, the temperature at the centre of a hot product drops much more slowly than the temperature at the surface.

If food has been deep frozen and thawed it must not be refrozen for the same reason. Bacteria are not often killed by deep freeze temperatures and when the food is thawed they will have a chance to multiply. If the food is then refrozen, a greatly increased number of bacteria will be present, all capable of multiplying next time it is thawed.

3. Cool food quickly and keep it cold until it is ready to be served or reheated

All foods should be cooled as quickly as possible so that harmful bacteria will have only a short time at a temperature at which they can multiply. Cooked food should not be taken straight from the oven and put into the refrigerator, however, as this will increase the temperature of the refrigerator to a dangerously high level, and food poisoning bacteria may be able to multiply in other foods being stored there.

Place hot cooked foods in a cold room or cool area of the kitchen and then put them in the refrigerator, e.g. within $1\frac{1}{2}$ hours. To speed up the cooling process, large volumes of meat can be divided and cooled in smaller containers.

4. Never keep food warm

Keep food either very hot or very cold. Do not keep it in a warm atmosphere, e.g. a service counter, as this will allow the rapid multiplication of bacteria. If food is to be served hot it should be served as soon as possible after cooking and provided the temperature is kept above 63 °C there is little danger of bacteria multiplying.

If food is to be served cold, it should be stored in a refrigerator until just before it is served.

These rules are particularly important if the food concerned is susceptible to bacterial growth e.g. meats and meat products, gravies, milk and cream products.

5. Never reheat food more than once

Reheating food is always a hazard because cooked food may still contain spores of *C. perfringens* or *B. cereus* or it may have been contaminated with any type of bacteria after cooking. When the food is cooled the spores will germinate and start to multiply along with any other bacteria present. When the food is warmed up, the temperatures used are not normally high enough to destroy toxins or to kill spore-forming bacteria.

If reheating is absolutely necessary, the food should be covered and cooled very rapidly after cooking and stored in a refrigerator until it is ready to be reheated. It should then be reheated rapidly and thoroughly. Hot gravy or sauce should never be added to cold food in order to heat it up, since the combined temperature will probably be optimum for bacterial growth.

Under no circumstances should meat products or rice be reheated more than once because each time a food is reheated there are two opportunities for bacteria to multiply, once during the heating up process and once during the cooling down process. In schools and hospitals the usual policy is not to reheat foods at all, since children and sick people are particularly susceptible to food poisoning.

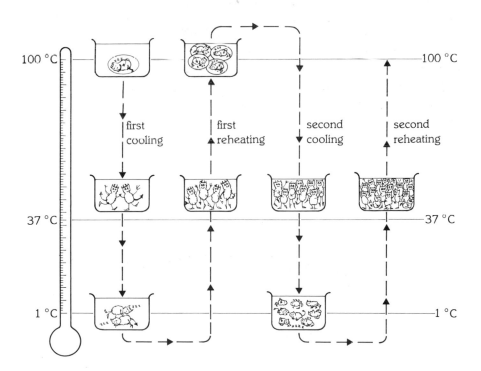

Factors contributing to 1479 outbreaks of food poisoning in England and Wales

Contributing factor	*Salmonella*	*C. perfringens*	*S. aureus*	*B. cereus*	*Other*	Total
Preparation too far in advance	240	464	80	54	6	844
Storage at ambient temperature	172	276	75	39	4	566
Inadequate cooling	125	313	12	17	1	468
Inadequate reheating	76	275	5	33	2	391
Contaminated processed food	100	19	27	4	86	236
Undercooking	139	74	2	1	7	223
Contaminated canned food	2	4	42	1	55	104
Inadequate thawing	61	34	—	—	—	95
Cross-contamination	84	8	2	—	—	94
Raw food consumed	84	—	1	—	8	93
Improper warm holding	15	52	—	8	2	77
Infected food handlers	13	—	50	—	2	65
Use of left overs	25	25	11	1	—	62
Extra large quantities prepared	29	17	2	—	—	48

Source: PHLS Communicable Disease Surveillance Centre
Extracted from Diane Roberts 'Factors contributing to outbreaks of food poisoning in England and Wales 1970-1979', The Journal of Hygiene, volume 89, 1982, pp 491-8. (updated) (Several factors may contribute to one outbreak.)

SUMMARY

1. All frozen meat should be thoroughly thawed before cooking.

2. Food must be kept either very hot or very cold before it is served and never left in a warm temperature for any length of time.

3. The practice of reheating food should be avoided wherever possible. Meat products and rice must never be reheated more than once.

Chapter 12

Temperature Control of Food

The previous chapter explained the importance of keeping food either very hot (above 63 °C) or very cold (below 8 °C). Most kitchens have refrigerators, freezers and sometimes cool rooms for low temperature storage and some means of keeping food very hot when it is about to be served. In addition, microwave ovens are frequently used to reheat foods quickly. The successful use of various combinations of this equipment will ensure that food spends very little time at a temperature at which bacteria will multiply.

REFRIGERATORS

Operating temperature

A refrigerator should operate at a temperature between 1 °C and 4 °C. Most food poisoning bacteria will not multiply at this temperature but they will not be killed. During refrigerated storage, food poisoning bacteria are usually dormant but as soon as the food is removed from the refrigerator and put in a warm room they will start to multiply rapidly. Many food spoilage bacteria are able to multiply in the refrigerator but at a much slower rate than at room temperature.

To maintain the correct temperature it is important to:

1. Keep the door shut whenever possible.

2. Cool hot foods before putting them in the refrigerator. Hot foods would cause a considerable increase in the temperature and also condensation which may lead to cross-contamination.

3. Defrost regularly. Defrosting is the removal of excess ice which forms around the refrigerating coils and reduces their efficiency.

The temperature of the refrigerator should not be allowed to drop below 1 °C because ice crystals would form in the food causing loss of texture and quality.

Position of foods

The position of foods in a refrigerator should be carefully planned so that cross-contamination will not occur. Raw meat, poultry, vegetables and fish should be stored separately from prepared food which will not be cooked again. If there is more than one refrigerator in the kitchen, different ones can be used for raw and cooked foods. If there is only one, raw foods should be stored at the bottom of the refrigerator and cooked foods at the top so that contaminated blood or food particles cannot drop from the raw foods to the cooked foods. Strong-smelling foods such as fish should be put in an airtight container and placed as far away as possible from foods which readily absorb smells, such as butter.

Covering of foods in the refrigerator prevents drying out, cross-contamination and the absorption of odours. Cling film is useful for this purpose but should not be placed over the food until it has cooled. The condensation which collects when cling film is placed over warm food speeds up spoilage of that food. Cling film should not be allowed to touch the food it is covering and so should not be used to wrap foods, particularly those which have a high fat content, e.g. cheese. The 'clinging' properties of cling film come from substances known as plasticisers present in the film. These plasticisers have been shown to migrate into fatty foods when the film is in direct contact with the food. In general, cling film that clings well contains more plasticisers than 'low migration' cling film, which clings less well. However, some migration will still take place from low migration film. The migration of plasticisers increases when the cling film is heated and for this reason it should not be used in contact with food in a microwave or conventional oven.

There is no definite evidence to suggest that the levels of plasticisers found in food that has been in contact with cling film are harmful, but until more research is done the above recommendations should be observed.

A refrigerator functions by circulating cold air round the food so it is essential that it is not so tightly packed that the circulation of air is restricted.

There have been many recent developments in refrigeration units for use in large catering establishments. The basic unit is the 'reach-in' cabinet which is available in many sizes. Any combination of removable internal fittings such as shelves or deep containers can be chosen depending on storage requirements. All these are removable to facilitate cleaning. Stainless steel doors are usually fitted to withstand tough treatment in busy kitchens.

For even larger quantities, 'roll-in' refrigerators are available which will accommodate trolleys of food. Some have a door at the preparations end and a door at the opposite end which opens in the serving area.

Other refrigeration units include mobile refrigerators for food which is to be served a distance from the preparation area and refrigerators with glass doors which can be used for displaying food such as cream cakes and wine. Refrigerators with glass doors must not be positioned so that the door is in direct sunlight because this allows heat to build up in the refrigerator in the same way as it does in a greenhouse.

CHILLERS

A refrigerator should not be used to cool hot food, and in a catering establishment where large volumes of food such as roast meats and poultry must be cooled quickly before refrigerating a blast chiller is almost essential. The temperature of the food is reduced quickly to 15 °C due to the circulation of a continuous current of cold air.

FREEZERS

Operating temperature

The length of time which food can be safely stored in a freezer depends on the temperature of the freezer. A star marking system has been devised which indicates the temperature of the freezer and consequently the time for which food may be stored.

Most domestic freezers operate at −18 °C and are capable of freezing fresh food without affecting the temperature of the frozen food already in the cabinet. Some bacteria will be killed during storage at this temperature but many can remain dormant for long periods of time. Spores and toxins are not affected by deep freezing. When food is taken out of the deep freeze and thawed, the surviving bacteria start to grow and multiply again. Food that has been frozen tends to allow more rapid bacterial growth than the equivalent fresh food and therefore deteriorates rather more quickly.

The star marking system for frozen food compartments

	temperature of freezer	food storage time
✳	−6 °C (21 °F)	1 week
✳✳	−12 °C (10 °F)	1 month
✳✳✳	−18 °C (0 °F)	3 months
✳✳✳✳	−18 °C (0 °F) to −25 °C (−15 °C)	3 months or longer; capable of freezing fresh food

Refreezing

Food should not be refrozen once it has thawed unless it is cooked in between. There are two reasons for this:

1. If the thawed food is kept at a temperature above 8 °C for some time, any pathogenic bacteria present will have a chance to multiply.

2. The texture of the food will suffer. Large ice crystals tend to form when food is frozen relatively slowly in domestic freezers. The loss of texture which this causes is more noticeable in food which has been thawed and refrozen.

Freezer breakdown

If there is a power cut or the freezer breaks down, the door or lid should be kept closed and covered with blankets to minimize the temperature increase. If the food is still partially frozen when the power is restored or the freezer is mended, it may be safe to refreeze the food. If in doubt, an environmental health officer will give advice on this matter. If the food has completely thawed out, one of the following options must be chosen:

1. Use the food immediately.

2. Store the food in a refrigerator but for no longer than 2 days.

3. Cook the food thoroughly, cool rapidly and store in a refrigerator for no longer than 3 days.

4. Destroy the food.

MICROWAVE OVENS

Microwave ovens provide a quick and convenient way of cooking and reheating food provided they are used correctly.

Any catering establishment that uses a microwave oven regularly for cooking or reheating should use a commercial model. Domestic microwave ovens have a life expectancy of 2000 hours and an output of between 500 and 700 watts, whereas commercial microwave ovens are designed to last for many more hours of use and have an output of between 700 and 1600 watts. Food can therefore be defrosted, cooked and reheated more efficiently in a commercial microwave oven.

In order to ensure that food cooked in a microwave oven does not cause food poisoning, the same principles that apply in conventional cooking must be followed.

1. Defrost food completely before starting to cook it.

2. Cook food thoroughly, by cooking it for the required length of time on the correct power setting. The temperature in the centre of the food must reach 70 °C for at least 2 minutes. The time required to reach this temperature will depend on the density and quantity of the food.

3. Observe standing times, as this is part of the cooking process.

4. Never reheat meat or rice, or foods containing them more than once.

It can be useful to make a table similar to the one below, which gives the correct cooking times and standing times, for the foods most frequently handled.

Food	Setting	Time	Standing time
Trout (6 oz)	Defrost	2½ min	1 min
Chicken joint (8 oz)	Defrost	3 min	2 min
Plated meal (16 oz)	Defrost	5½ min	2 min
Frozen sandwich	Defrost	1½ min	30 sec
Meat pie (5 oz)	Heating	25 sec	30 sec
Meat pie (5 oz) × 5	Heating	1¼ min	1 min
Plated meal (16 oz)	Heating	1½ min	1 min
Apple pie — 8 portions	Heating	3½ min	1 min
Pizza (8 in)	Heating	40 sec	30 sec
Pizza (8 in) × 4	Heating	60 sec	1 min
Chicken (3 lb 6 oz)	Cooking	16 min	3 min
Trout (6 oz)	Cooking	1 min	30 sec
Frozen peas (2 lb)	Cooking	4½ min	—

Microwave ovens should be cleaned regularly, in particularly around the door seal because the presence of dirt and grease may stop the door closing correctly. They should be checked every year to ensure there is no leakage of microwaves. Local Environmental Health Departments often provide a testing service.

HOLDING UNITS

Many kitchens have a hot cupboard and/or a *bain-marie* for keeping food warm for short periods of time just before it is served. A hot cupboard is heated by gas or electricity and a *bain-marie* is a heated well filled with hot water. Both systems should be hot enough to ensure that the temperature at the centre of the food is kept above 63 °C. They must never be used for heating up cold foods as the process would be too slow using either piece of equipment.

COOK-CHILL AND COOK-FREEZE SYSTEMS

These methods of food preparation are becoming increasingly common and are widely used where centralised catering is practised. The food usually has to be transported a long distance from the kitchens where it is prepared, e.g. aeroplane meals, school meals, hospital meals. In any of these situations it would be unsatisfactory to cook the food and keep it warm untll it is required.

In cook-chill and cook-freeze systems the food is prepared in the central preparation unit: it is cooked thoroughly and then divided into individual portions observing strict hygiene standards. All containers are marked with the date (to ensure effective stock rotation) and also with the contents, reheating time and any other instructions.

Cook-chill   The food is chilled in a blast chiller to between 1 °C and 3 °C within two hours of cooking and must be kept in a refrigerator at this temperature until it is required for distribution. It should be reheated within two hours of arrival at the point of consumption. The temperature in the centre of the food must reach 70 °C for at least two minutes. All meals must be eaten within five days including the day of preparation. There is no danger of cook-chill foods causing food poisoning if these conditions are met.

A bacterium called *Listeria monocytogenes* (see p. 121) is found in approximately twenty per cent of cook-chill meals. It only grows slowly at refrigeration temperatures but it is important to observe the storage instructions, the 'eat by' date on the cover and the heating instructions. The bacterium does not form a spore and thorough heating of the meal all the way through will ensure that is safe to eat. Great care must be taken to ensure thorough and uniform heating if cook-chill meals are reheated in a microwave. The food must be cooked for the required length of time on the stated power setting and in the correct position. Instructions for standing times must also be observed because the food is continuing to cook by conduction during this period.

Cook-freeze   The food is blast-frozen (a very rapid method of freezing) to a temperature of −18 °C and kept at this temperature until required.

When it is reheated, the temperature in the centre of the food must reach 70 °C for at least two minutes.

Whichever system is used, any reheated food which is not consumed must be discarded.

It is important to bear in mind that any departure from these guidelines could result in an outbreak of food poisoning involving a large number of people. Further details can be obtained from the DoH code of practice *Guidelines on pre-cooked chilled foods*.

DATE-MARKING

Food labelling regulations introduced on 1st January 1991 made it compulsory for most foods to carry a date-mark. The date-mark on a food is the date before which the food should be eaten. If the food has been stored correctly it will be fresh and safe to eat on this date but the quality cannot be guaranteed beyond it.

The date-mark can be in one of three forms:

For foods that keep for 3 months or less
'BEST BEFORE' followed by the day and month.

For foods that keep for more than 3 months
'BEST BEFORE END' followed by the month and year.

For highly perishable foods, that is, those likely to cause illness if not eaten in the recommended time
'USE BY' followed by the day and month.

It is an offence to sell food for consumption after the 'use by' date.

Any special storage conditions necessary should appear after each date mark e.g. 'store in a refrigerator'.

SUMMARY

1. The temperature of a refrigerator must be maintained between 1 °C and 4 °C.

2. Frozen food should not be refrozen once it has thawed.

3. Microwave ovens provide a quick method of cooking and reheating food.

4. Holding units must not be used for heating up cold foods.

5. The cook-chill and cook-freeze methods of food preparation are useful when food has to be cooked some distance from where it is to be served.

Chapter 13

Foods Most Likely to Cause Food Poisoning

Some foods favour the growth of food poisoning bacteria; others do not.

When food poisoning is confirmed it is not always easy to identify the food which has caused the outbreak as there are frequently no samples of the suspected foods left. However, certain foods are regarded as being 'high-risk' and, if eaten just before the illness, will be suspected as the cause. In some of the investigated outbreaks sufficient evidence is available to implicate one particular food.

Analysis of 1562 outbreaks of food poisoning

Food vehicle	Salmonella sp	Clostridium perfringens	Staphylococcus aureus	Bacillus cereus	Total
Chicken	51	19	2	3	75
Turkey	28	11	1	1	41
Poultry	3	1	—	—	4
Beef	5	21	4	1	31
Pork/ham	18	17	5	1	41
Lamb/mutton	1	3	—	—	4
Mixed and other meats, pies and sausages	36	35	3	6	80
Gravy/sauces	—	3	—	—	3
Milk/cream	13	—	—	—	13
Eggs	44	—	3	1	48
Pasta dishes	2	4	—	1	7
Rice	1	—	—	13	14
Shellfish/fish	6	1	2	1	10
Other mixed foods	18	12	10	27	67
Not known	1089	32	—	3	1124
Total	1315	159	30	58	1562

Source: PHLS Communicable Disease Surveillance Centre

HIGH-RISK FOODS

Foods which encourage the growth of bacteria are usually high in protein and moisture. Examples are meat, poultry, eggs, milk and any foods where these are ingredients. Special precautions must be taken when preparing high-risk foods to ensure that:

1. They are not contaminated during preparation especially if they will be eaten uncooked or after only gently heating.

2. They are not left in a warm temperature for any longer than is absolutely necessary for their preparation so that there will be little time for any bacteria present to multiply. They should be served hot (above 63 °C) or cold (straight from the refrigerator).

MEAT AND MEAT PRODUCTS

Every year the majority of food poisoning outbreaks are caused by meat and meat products.

Freshly roasted meat

Freshly roasted or grilled meat, served hot immediately after cooking, is rarely a cause of food poisoning. Even a rare steak is safe because bacteria are not present in the centre of the meat, only on the surface.

Chickens

It is estimated that 70 per cent of raw chickens carry *Salmonella*. However, freshly roasted chickens or other poultry will cause food poisoning only if they have been cooked for less than the recommended time or if they were not completely defrosted before cooking.

Rolled joints

Rolled joints are more frequently a cause of food poisoning because surface meat which may be contaminated will be at the centre of the joint after rolling and also considerable handling by the chef is necessary. It is therefore essential that rolled joints should be small enough to allow sufficient heat to kill bacteria to penetrate to the centre during cooking.

Cold meats

Cold meats are frequently a cause of food poisoning usually because they have been contaminated after cooking and kept in a warm environment for several hours before serving.

Stews and casseroles

If served hot immediately after cooking, stews and casseroles will not cause food poisoning If they are kept warm for several hours or cooled slowly and reheated the next day, there is far more chance that they will cause food poisoning because any spores of C. perfringens which survived the first cooking process will have had time to germinate and multiply.

Minced meat

When meat is minced, any pathogenic bacteria which were present on the surface are distributed throughout the mass of the meat. Only sufficient meat to provide a day's supply should be minced at any one time.

Pies, pasties, rissoles, sausages and other 'made-up' meat dishes

'Made-up' meat dishes are frequently a cause of food poisoning because bacteria may be present throughout the food. Care must be taken to cook sufficiently to kill any bacteria in the centre.

Stocks

Stocks and gravies, soups and sauces made from them are an ideal medium for bacterial growth. They should be kept either hot (above 63 °C) until they are served or cold (below 8 °C) until they are reheated for service. If they are kept warm for several hours before being reheated for service, they are a likely cause of food poisoning.

Gelatin

Powdered gelatin frequently contains dormant food poisoning bacteria. When it is melted in water for use in meat pies or as a glaze it becomes an ideal food for bacterial growth and must therefore be kept at a temperature above 63 °C until it is used.

FISH

Freshly cooked fish is rarely a cause of food poisoning because food poisoning bacteria are not usually present in the intestines of cold-blooded animals. Shellfish have been known to cause food poisoning because they have been gathered from polluted waters but there are strict laws governing the gathering and cleansing of them. Fish dishes such as fish cakes or fish pie may be contaminated during preparation and should therefore always be stored correctly and reheated thoroughly.

DAIRY PRODUCTS

Milk

Most milk for sale in this country has been pasteurised which means that it is free of pathogenic bacteria. However, milk is an ideal food for bacterial growth and could cause food poisoning if contaminated after pasteurisation. Any dishes where milk is an ingredient, such as custards, trifles, milk puddings and sauces, must be served hot or refrigerated until served. Raw (unpasteurised) milk sometimes causes outbreaks of food poisoning.

Cream

Cream for sale in this country has been pasteurised. Cream, like milk, is an ideal food for bacterial growth if it is contaminated after pasteurisation. All cream cakes, trifles etc. should be kept cold until just before they are served. The same precautions must be taken with imitation cream.

Evaporated milk

Evaporated milk is safe when the can is first opened but supports the growth of bacteria and if not used straight away should be stored in the refrigerator.

Condensed milk

The high sugar content of condensed milk makes it unsuitable for bacterial growth.

Dried milk

Dried milk powder contains many dormant bacteria. Once reconstituted it must be treated as fresh milk and stored in the refrigerator.

Ice cream

Ice cream purchased from a reputable supplier can be regarded as safe. Ice cream should not be thawed and then refrozen.

Cheese

In Britain, cheese is normally made from pasteurised milk and is therefore rarely a cause of food poisoning. Hard cheeses do not contain sufficient moisture for bacterial growth, but low-fat cheeses do and can be a cause of food poisoning. Soft ripened cheeses such as Brie and Camembert are made from unpasteurised milk and are frequently contaminated with *Listeria* (see p. 121).

EGGS

Raw egg is ideal for bacterial growth. A small proportion of hen eggs carry *Salmonella* inside the shell. It is therefore preferable to cook eggs thoroughly, especially if they are to be eaten by an elderly, very young or sick person, since these people would be more seriously affected by food poisoning. Eggs should be stored in a refrigerator and any cracked eggs should not be used. Pasteurised liquid egg and dried egg are available as safer alternatives to raw egg.

Duck eggs are more frequently contaminated with *Salmonella* inside the shell and should always be thoroughly cooked.

Egg shells are often contaminated so care must be taken to prevent the transfer of bacteria from the shell to other food in the kitchen.

RICE

Rice is often contaminated with *B. cereus* which forms spores capable of surviving the cooking process. If rice is not eaten immediately after cooking it must be stored in the refrigerator.

LOW-RISK FOODS

Certain foods do not normally cause food poisoning because they do not provide bacteria with the nutrients they require for growth and multiplication. Foods with a high concentration of sugar, salt, acid or fat or dry foods will not support the growth of food poisoning bacteria. (See Food Preservation pp. 109 and 110.)

Jams, syrup, honey, salted meat

These foods are unlikely to cause food poisoning because the sugar/salt concentration is too high. The sugar and salt present in the food dissolve in the water to form a concentrated solution leaving insufficient moisture for bacterial growth.

Fatty foods

Very few types of bacteria can multiply in the presence of high concentrations of fat and those which can are not the ones that cause food poisoning.

Acid foods

Food poisoning bacteria will not grow in very acid foods such as pickles and citrus fruits.

Dry foods

Dry foods will not support the growth of food poisoning bacteria but may contain them. If water is added at a later stage in preparation the bacteria will be able to multiply again so the food must then be treated as fresh food and stored in a refrigerator.

Canned foods

In Britain, food is canned and sterilised under strict control and any manufactured canned food can be regarded as safe unless the can is damaged. If it is punctured, has a faulty seam or swollen ends (caused by gas produced inside the can) the manufacturer should be notified and the can and contents either returned or thrown away. Canned ham is often pasteurised only, since sterilisation affects the quality of the ham; it must therefore be stored in a refrigerator. After canned food has been opened it should be handled and stored as fresh food.

SUMMARY

1. Moist, high protein foods will usually support the growth of food poisoning bacteria.
2. Foods with a high concentration of sugar, salt, acid or fat or dry foods will not support the growth of food poisoning bacteria.

Chapter 14

How Common is Food Poisoning?

The number of reported cases of food poisoning is showing an increase in most years despite higher standards of hygiene and increased awareness of the causes of food poisoning. Notified food poisoning cases in England and Wales more than doubled between 1985 and 1990 and the total continues to increase. It is estimated that there are at least ten times as many cases which are not reported and are therefore not included in these figures.

Reported cases of bacterial food poisoning

1980	1985	1990	1991	1992	1993	1994
10318	13143	36945	35291	42551	44271	50692

Source: Public Health Laboratory Service Communicable Disease Surveillance Centre

There are a number of reasons for this increase:

1. Intensive rearing of farm animals such as chickens and pigs. The concentrated feeds which are given to them are frequently contaminated with *Salmonella*, and because the animals are so crowded, bacteria can easily spread from one to another. The meat we buy is therefore often contaminated with pathogenic bacteria.

2. The practice of eating out is becoming far more popular and the
    majority of the working population is eating at least one meal a day
    in a restaurant, pub or canteen. If a mistake is made in food
    preparation in one of these catering establishments a large number
    of people will be affected, whereas a similar incident in the home
    will affect only a small number of people.

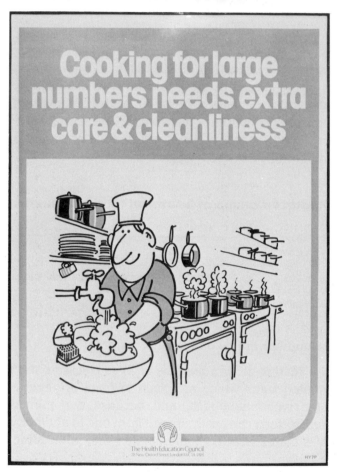

Health Education Council poster

3. Restaurants, canteens etc. produce a much more varied range of
    dishes than used to be the case. With this degree of choice, instead
    of food being served hot immediately after it is cooked, there is
    tendency to keep foods warm until a customer requests a particular
    dish. The increasing use of microwave ovens will hopefully reduce
    cases of food poisoning caused by keeping food warm.

~~~~~~~ MENU ~~~~~~~

Chilli con carne	2·70
Hungarian goulash	2·65
Moussaka	2·90
Sweet and sour pork	3·00
Lasagne	2·80
Chicken and prawn pilaff	3·10
Beef and mushroom pie	2·75
Spaghetti bolognese	2·75

———————//———————

Black Forest gâteau	1·75
Sherry trifle	1·75
Chocolate mousse	1·50

4. There has been a rapid growth in the number of shops selling take-away meals. The food is frequently cooked in advance and then reheated on purchase. If it is not cooled quickly and stored in a refrigerator between cooking and reheating there will be plenty of opportunity for bacterial growth.

TAKE-AWAY MENU

Chicken and chips	2.30	Lamb curry and rice	2.75
Steak pie and chips	1.50	Beef curry and rice	2.85
Cheeseburger	2.20	Special fried rice	2.20
Pizza	2.35	Sweet and sour pork	3.00
Barbecued spare ribs	2.95	Sweet and sour chicken	2.95
Jacket potato		Doner kebab	2.30
– with chicken	2.00	Shish kebab	2.40
– with prawns	2.20		

SERVED WITHIN 5 MINUTES OF ORDERING

5. Large-scale factory production of foods has led to an increase in food poisoning. Although factory processes are normally very carefully controlled, a slight error at some stage in production could lead to thousands of contaminated prepacked foods which may be distributed throughout the country.

6. Many housewives now work full-time, hence shopping is probably done weekly rather than daily, resulting in a greater chance of bacterial growth in the food after purchase unless it is stored correctly. Meals are sometimes cooked ahead of requirements and reheated when needed which increases the chance for bacterial growth.

7. The majority of outbreaks of food poisoning occur during the summer months. In the summer, there is an increased tendency to pack foods, e.g. for picnics and for journeys to holiday resorts. These are often kept at warm temperatures for several hours before they are eaten. Insulated bags and ice boxes should be used to keep food cool if it will not be eaten for several hours after removal from the refrigerator. Flies present a hygiene problem in the summer months.

8. Untrained staff are often employed during the summer months to cope with the increased demand for restaurant meals. All staff should be taught the basic principles of food hygiene and should be carefully supervised in their first few weeks' work.

SUMMARY

1. The number of cases of food poisoning is increasing in most years due to:
    (a) Intensive rearing of farm animals.
    (b) An increased tendency to eat out.
    (c) A much more varied menu.
    (d) An increasing number of shops selling take-away meals.
    (e) Large scale factory production of food.
    (f) An increased tendency to shop and cook several days in advance of eating.

2. The majority of outbreaks of food poisoning occur in the summer months.

3. It is very important for all food handlers to be trained in food hygiene.

Chapter 15

Washing-up

The aim of washing-up is to remove visible food waste and to destroy bacteria. It is very important that all utensils, crockery containers, etc. used for food should be thoroughly cleaned and disinfected each time they are used. Kitchen equipment that is not clean is likely to contaminate food that subsequently comes into contact with it.

Cleaning removes grease and dirt. Hot water and detergent are normally used to clean kitchen equipment.

Disinfection removes vegetative bacteria, but not spores. Disinfection can be achieved by the use of very hot water on its own or by the use of chemicals.

Sterilisation removes all bacteria and their spores. Sterilisation can be achieved by the use of steam or chemicals.

THE NEED FOR DISINFECTION

It is not necessary to sterilise equipment used for food preparation: disinfecting it is adequate.

Some surfaces and equipment in a kitchen do not even need to be disinfected, for example floors and walls; a detergent wash is sufficient. Disinfection after cleaning is normally considered necessary for:

1. Work surfaces in direct contact with food.

2. The hands of the food handler.

3. Equipment touched by the food handler during preparation, e.g. refrigerator door handles.

4. Cleaning materials and equipment.

DETERGENTS

Detergents are chemicals that when added to water, help to remove grease, dirt and food residues.

A detergent does not kill bacteria but reduces the number present on an article by removing the dirt and grease that harbour them. If water without detergent is used on a greasy surface, the water tends to form droplets and will not remove the food residues effectively. Detergents are most effective when used with hot water.

Stage I

Water does not spread evenly on greasy plates and tends to form small droplets

Stage II

The water now spreads on the grease;
The detergent molecules 'fasten' the water and grease together;
Rubbing with a cloth or sponge removes grease and dirt together from the plate.

Stage III

Detergent is added to the water;
The detergent molecules surround the water droplets;
The head of the molecule (water-loving end) enters the water;
The tail (water-hating end) is attracted to the grease.

Stage IV

Grease droplet

Water

The grease now rolls up into drops surrounded by detergent molecules and is suspended in the water. When the water goes down the drain the grease goes with it.

Washing-up liquid is a detergent used in the home and in industrial kitchens to clean utensils and most equipment. Its action is fairly mild and other detergents are available for heavily soiled equipment. A very alkaline detergent is used in dishwashers and can be used for removing baked-on grease from kitchen equipment.

DISINFECTANTS

The best method of disinfecting kitchen equipment is to immerse it in very hot water (80–88 °C) for two to three minutes. This method should be used whenever possible, but if it is not practicable a chemical disinfectant can be used. The ones most commonly used in catering premises contain either hypochlorites or iodophors as the active ingredient.

Hypochlorites are inexpensive and provided they are used at the correct dilution, are very effective and leave little taste or smell. For disinfection they must be left in contact with the equipment for a specific time, called the 'contact time'. The main disadvantage of hypochlorites is that they are easily inactivated by food particles and so are only effective when the equipment has already been thoroughly cleaned with hot water and a detergent.

Iodophors disinfect surfaces rapidly, leaving little taste and smell, but again are easily inactivated by food residues. Cleaning materials containing iodophors tend to be more expensive than those containing hypochlorites.

SANITISERS

Sanitisers are chemicals which combine both a detergent and disinfectant. Chemical disinfectants are partially inactivated by dirt and food residues, so sanitisers are not as effective for dirty equipment and surfaces as a detergent wash followed by disinfection. They are suitable for lightly soiled equipment or surfaces.

WASHING-UP PROCEDURE

Washing-up should not take place in a food preparation area because of the danger of dirty plates contaminating work surfaces which are to be used for the preparation of food. If a kitchen serves a canteen or restaurant, the washing-up area should be next to the restaurant so that dirty crockery and utensils need not be brought into the food preparation area at all. Washing up can be done either by hand, in which case at least two sinks are necessary, or by a dish-washing machine. Whichever method is used, the process is similar and comprises three stages.

1. *Preparation* Crockery should be scraped clean and if possible all crockery and utensils should be given a pre-rinse in warm water so that the washing water at the next stage will stay cleaner.

2. *Main wash* At this stage a detergent is added to the water to help remove food remains and grease.
    The temperature of the water should be between 50 °C and 60 °C. This is too hot for bare hands so rubber gloves will be needed. It should not exceed 63 °C because certain protein residues such as traces of egg become baked on to plates and cutlery if water hotter than this is used. Wiping with a clean nylon brush or a disposable dishcloth in this combination of hot water and detergent will remove grease and food residues but it will not make the equipment completely free from bacteria.
    The washing-up water must be changed frequently and more detergent added so it will always be both clean and at the correct temperature.

3. *Rinsing stage* The articles are transferred from the sink which contains water and detergent into a sink containing very hot water

at a temperature of about 80 °C. They are left immersed in the water for 2 minutes. The purpose of this stage is:

(a) to rinse off any traces of detergent;
(b) to kill any remaining bacteria;
(c) to heat the articles to a sufficiently high temperature to allow them to air dry.

This disinfection process will only be performed effectively if the temperature is maintained at 80 °C. If this is not possible, a chemical disinfectant should be added to the rinsing water to destroy the bacteria which are still present after the detergent wash.

Nutrient agar plate showing bacteria present
in one drop of liquid from a dirty dishcloth

4. *Drying* It is generally considered best to allow crockery and utensils to drain dry in racks. They will dry fairly quickly if the temperature of the rinse water is maintained at 80 °C. Clean, dry crockery and utensils should be stored under cover so that they will not be re-contaminated.

Nutrient agar plates showing bacteria present on a chopping board after preparing raw meat

Without washing

After wiping with a dishcloth

After correct washing-up

GUIDELINES FOR THE USE OF CLEANING CHEMICALS

1. Store chemicals away from food, preferably in a cool, dry storeroom.
2. Store chemical containers in an upright position and firmly closed.
3. Ensure all containers are labelled correctly. Never use empty food or drink containers for storing chemicals because of the risk of a mistake being made.
4. Follow the manufacturer's instructions about dilution rates. A solution that is too strong may damage surfaces, one that is too weak will be ineffective.
5. Make a fresh solution at least daily.
6. Do not leave cloths, mops or brushes in a disinfectant solution which has been used. The dirt will inactivate the disinfectant and the cleaning equipment will become a breeding ground for micro-organisms.

Dish-washing machines

There are many different types of dish-washing machines all of which vary slightly in their operation. It is therefore important to follow the manufacturer's instructions. The principle is the same as for the hand-washing method. Dirty crockery and utensils are stacked into the machine, pre-rinsed, washed in water at 60 °C and a detergent, and then rinsed at a temperature between 80 °C and 88 °C. They should be allowed to air-dry under cover.

It is essential that regular checks are made to ensure that the dish-washing machine is working correctly. Most industrial machines have dials on the outside so that the operator can check that the temperatures of the water are correct and that the articles are exposed to the very hot rinsing water for the correct length of time.

Glassware

Glassware should be washed by a two-stage method with detergent and water at 50–60 °C in the first sink and water at 80 °C in the second sink. If the glassware will not stand this temperature, a chemical disinfectant must be added to the second sink. Small glass-washing machines which can be fixed to the bar itself are often used in licensed premises. A sanitiser is added to the water and the cleaning action is performed by revolving brushes whilst the glass is held in place by hand. Machines with a separate rinsing chamber are preferable to single-chamber machines.

Glass-washing machine

The pan-wash

Pots, pans and other cooking vessels should be washed separately from crockery and cutlery. A tap proportioner can be fitted which will draw the correct amount of detergent from a container and mix it with the water. Scouring pads should be available. Stubborn grease can be removed by adding an alkali such as washing soda (sodium bicarbonate).

Tap proportioner

Working surfaces

Working surfaces should be cleaned as follows:

1. Wipe off crumbs and loose dirt.

2. Wash down with a detergent and water at a temperature of 50–60 °C using a disposable cloth.

3. Rinse thoroughly with a chemical disinfectant added to the water. This disinfectant solution must remain in contact with the surface for the time recommended in the instructions. Sanitisers (a detergent combined with a disinfectant) can be used for surfaces that are visibly clean, in which case stages 2 and 3 are combined.

Other equipment

A cleaning routine should be established for all large articles of equipment in use in the kitchen. As a general rule, all equipment which comes into direct contact with food should be cleaned after every use. Other surfaces and equipment should be cleaned as necessary. To ensure that cleaning is not overlooked it is a good idea to draw up a cleaning schedule which lists the items to be cleaned, the frequency and method of cleaning and the name of the person to whom the task is allotted.

HYGIENE SCHEDULE

All electrical appliances must be switched off and disconnected

Frequency	Item	Method	Product	Allotted to
	Refrigerators and cold storage rooms	Clean all surfaces with a detergent and hot water followed by a disinfectant solution. Rinse with clean water and air-dry.		
	Floors	Apply detergent solution with clean string mop. Rinse. Air-dry.		
	Walls, doors and paintwork	Spray or sponge surfaces with detergent solution. Wipe clean with fresh, moist cloth		
	Boilers and steamers	Scrub all surfaces with detergent. Rinse and air-dry. To descale: use recommended descaler. Rinse and air-dry.		
	Canopies	Spray or wipe surfaces with recommended detergent. Rinse and air-dry.		
	Tea/coffee urns	Scrub with recommended cleaning solution. Rinse thoroughly. Air-dry.		

Authorised by ....

Date ....

DISH-WASHING AT HOME

Few people have two sinks or a dish-washing machine at home so washing-up is not as conveniently done as in a large industrial kitchen. The temperatures used for washing with detergent and rinsing should be the same as in commercial premises. Rubber gloves will therefore be needed. After use, rubber gloves should be cleaned and dried.

It is important to remember that clean crockery and utensils can easily be recontaminated by a dirty tea towel. If tea towels are used for drying, it is essential that they are washed after each use. If the crockery and utensils are left to dry in the air they should be stacked away under cover as soon as they are dry and certainly before preparation and cooking of food begins again.

SUMMARY

1. Detergents remove dirt and grease but do not kill bacteria.

2. Disinfectants remove the majority of bacteria on surfaces and equipment.

3. Washing-up can be done by hand or machine. In both cases the articles to be cleaned are subjected to a detergent wash and are then rinsed in either hot water or water containing a chemical disinfectant.

4. Crockery and utensils should be covered and allowed to drain dry.

5. Glassware and pots and pans should be washed separately from the main wash.

6. Surfaces and equipment in contact with food should be cleaned and disinfected after use.

7. A cleaning schedule should be established for large equipment.

Chapter 16

Kitchen Design

It would be unrealistic for anyone to think that a kitchen can be made free from bacteria but there are several general principles concerning kitchen design and the layout of equipment which will help to reduce the risk of cross-contamination of foods. Apart from looking unpleasant, food crumbs, spillage from cooking, grease and dirt splashed on walls and on the floor, condensation on the ceiling and dust on window sills and floors will all be likely sources of pathogenic bacteria.

The main consideration in designing a kitchen is that the layout should allow easy cleaning and a continuous workflow from receiving raw foods through preparation and cooking to final presentation. Equipment should be movable or should be placed where it is possible to clean at the back, sides and underneath as well as at the front. If the equipment is not movable, it should, where possible, be built-in with one continuous surface between the equipment and the wall or floor so that dirt and grease cannot lodge in joints and corners.

A spacious kitchen is easier to keep clean and run hygienically than a small cramped kitchen. In a kitchen serving a restaurant, there must always be a division of preparation areas with the following points in mind:

1. Vegetable storage and preparation should be near to the delivery door. Potatoes and other vegetables have soil on them which carries *C. perfringens* spores and, if the vegetables are carried through the kitchen, dust from the vegetables may easily settle on cooked food.

2. Sections for raw meat preparation and cooked food preparation should be well separated to avoid cross-contamination because raw meat is frequently contaminated with *Salmonella* and *C. perfringens* bacteria.

3. The washing-up area should not be near the preparation areas so that dirty crockery and food waste will not come into contact with food to be eaten.

91

LIGHTING

In all kitchens it is essential that there is adequate lighting.

Natural light is less strain on the eyes than artificial light so windows should be large. Artificial light will of course be needed at times and should be bright enough to prevent accidents happening during food preparation and should be shadow-free so that all dirt is readily visible and the kitchen can be cleaned properly.

VENTILATION

Adequate ventilation in a kitchen is very important for two reasons:

1. To keep the temperature and humidity down. (The temperature and humidity of a hot steamy kitchen are ideal for bacterial growth.)

2. To remove cooking smells, steam, grease, etc.

    In a large industrial kitchen, hoods connected to extractor fans are usually fitted over the cookers. These must be cleaned regularly because grease and dirt reduce their efficiency.

    Windows which are opened for ventilation should be screened to prevent entry of insects and birds.

WORKING SURFACES

Working surfaces should be made from a hard-wearing easily cleaned material which will not absorb moisture, chip or crack, and will not be affected by food residues. Stainless steel is the usual choice. Wooden working surfaces should not be present as these rapidly become contaminated and are difficult to clean. Hardwood is still used for chopping boards but laminated plastic or compressed rubber boards are preferable. Different chopping boards must be used for preparing raw food and cooked food so that cross-contamination will not occur. Any surface which is chipped, cracked or badly scratched should be replaced as damaged surfaces will harbour food residues and hence bacteria.

WASTE DISPOSAL

Food waste is ideal for the growth of bacteria and unless it is carefully protected it will attract flies, rats, mice and other pests which may then transfer the bacteria back to fresh food in the kitchen.

Left-over food and residues from food preparation should be removed from the working area immediately and put into pedal bins lined with plastic sacks. Disposable paper sacks with pedal-operated metal lids can be used for dry waste. There should be an adequate number of bins in the kitchen so that waste does not have to be carried across the kitchen. The bins must never be allowed to overflow and should be emptied regularly at the end of the day even if not full in order to remove a source of food for pests. It is essential to wash the hands after handling refuse and before handling food again.

Paper sack with pedal-operated lid

A special area outside and not too near the kitchen window should be set aside for bins containing refuse and awaiting disposal. They should have tight fitting lids so that they cannot be knocked off by animals or blown off by the wind. An uncovered dustbin will attract flies and other pests. The bins should have rounded corners to facilitate cleaning and be placed on a metal stand approximately one foot above a drained and concreted area which should be washed down frequently. Alternatively, large heavy duty wheeled bins can be used.

Dustbins — correct type and storage

Waste disposal units

These are a modern and convenient way of dealing with waste. They are made up of a system of high-speed cutters which shred the waste food which is then washed away into the drainage system.

Food waste disposal unit

WASHING FACILITIES

An adequate number of hand-washing basins with hot and cold water, soap, a nailbrush and drying facilities must be present in convenient positions, e.g. at the entrance to the kitchen and next to the preparation areas. These must not be used for food preparation.

Stainless steel sinks should be located in each preparation area for washing food and must not be used for washing hands.

FLOORS

Kitchen floors should be made of a hard-wearing, anti-slip, easily cleaned material which will not absorb moisture and will not be affected by food residues such as grease, salt and fruit acids. Non-slip quarry tiles laid in acid-resisting cement and thick, non-slip vinyl sheets are both suitable. There should be no breaks or cracks in the surface as these will allow dirt and bacteria to accumulate. The junction of the floor with the wall should be coved (rounded).

CEILINGS

Ceilings should have a smooth finish to facilitate cleaning. Stove-enamelled metal tiles or plasterboard sheeting coved to the wall is suitable. Polystyrene tiles are unsuitable because of the fire risk and because they are difficult to clean.

WALLS

Walls should have smooth surfaces which will be easy to clean and should be light-coloured to make dirt easily visible. Areas which frequently become soiled, e.g. around sinks and cooking apparatus, are best covered with either stainless steel sheets or ceramic tiles. Areas less susceptible to splashing (above 1.5 m/5 ft) can be painted with a steam-resistant emulsion.

SUMMARY

1. A well-planned, easily cleaned kitchen will save time and effort in food preparation and will reduce the risk of contamination of food.

2. The kitchen must be well lit and ventilated.

3. Floors, walls and working surfaces should be made from smooth, hard-wearing and non-absorbent materials.

4. An adequate number of hand-washing basins and food preparation sinks must be present.

5. Waste disposal units or disposable plastic or paper sacks which are removed from the kitchen regularly are the most hygienic methods of waste disposal.

Chapter 17

Kitchen Pests

Rats, mice, flies and cockroaches are the most common kitchen pests. Clean, well constructed and well maintained premises will not harbour any of these pests and it is therefore the duty of the food handler to make the premises where he works unattractive to pests by maintaining a high standard of hygiene and by keeping buildings in good repair.

RATS AND MICE

When rats and mice infest kitchens they are capable of causing considerable damage to food by gnawing through packets of food in storage and by eating almost any food which is easily accessible to them. The main problem is not the quantity of food pests eat but the amount they contaminate with harmful bacteria. Rats and mice frequently carry *Salmonella* in their intestines and so their droppings will contain live bacteria. They also carry bacteria on their fur and feet and can therefore transfer food poisoning bacteria from soil, waste food and refuse to uncovered food and surfaces used for food preparation just by running over them. Rats sometimes carry the bacterium that causes Weil's disease, an illness which gives rise to jaundice and can be fatal.

Rats and mice often gnaw woodwork, water pipes and electrical cables in order to wear down their continually growing incisor teeth. They have been known to cause fires and floods and often make costly repairs necessary.

Rats and mice live and breed in warm dark corners where they will not be disturbed and where food is plentiful and easily accessible. To prevent infestation, food premises should be kept in good repair with no holes in the building and no defective pipes or drains. Pipe runs should be sealed at the entrance to buildings and wherever they pass from room to room.

Store rooms should be cleaned regularly. All stock must be kept off the ground and used in rotation to ensure that rats and mice are not being sheltered at the back of the store room.

Food should never be left uncovered in a kitchen and rubbish must not be allowed to accumulate inside or outside the building. All bins should have tight-fitting lids.

If any of the signs which indicate rodent infestation are noticed, such as gnawing marks, droppings or feet marks in dust or grain, measures to control it must be taken immediately because rodents breed prolifically. About 200 rats can develop from a pair and their young in a year, and given favourable conditions a pair of mice and their young can increase to 2000.

In the event of an infestation of rats or mice expert advice and treatment must be sought. The environmental health officer or a specialist organisation such as Rentokil should be contacted. Rats and mice are usually eliminated with poisons (rodenticides) which are laid in tamper-resistant bait boxes. Rats are very suspicious animals and baiting is necessary for at least two weeks before they will take the poisoned food. The 1986 Control of Pesticides Regulations strictly control the pesticides that may be used in food premises.

Brown rats

House mice

HOUSEFLIES AND BLUEBOTTLES

The number of flies in an urban environment has decreased significantly due to more efficient disposal of refuse and sewage but the fly is still a common pest in summer months. It feeds on refuse, from which it flies to human food where it deposits bacteria from its legs, wings, saliva and excrement.

Houseflies

Flies breed very rapidly. They lay their eggs in warm, moist places such as on waste food and refuse. At summer temperatures it takes only ten days for the egg to develop into a maggot and then into an adult fly.

Bluebottles are characterised by their large size, their blue colour and the buzzing noise they make whilst flying. They are attracted to meat and fish products on which they lay their eggs.

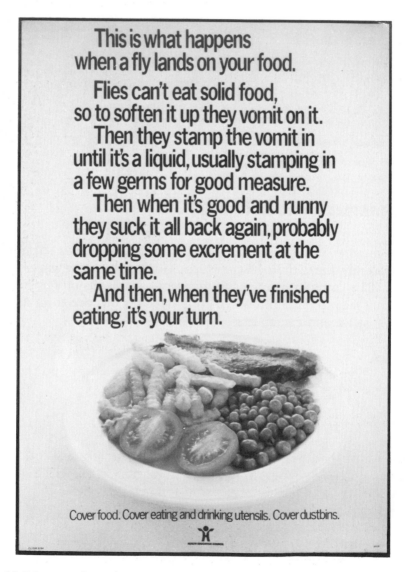

Health Education Council poster

The most effective method of reducing the number of flies in a kitchen is to cover windows, door spaces and ventilators with a gauze which is too fine to allow their entry. The use of mechanical waste disposal units also helps. If conventional bins are used, they should be kept firmly covered and regularly emptied and cleaned.

Insecticidal sprays must not be allowed to come into contact with food and therefore must not be used in rooms where food is prepared. Electrically operated fly killers are suitable for food preparation areas. They consist of an ultraviolet light which attracts flies to a metal grid with an electric current running through it. The flies are electrocuted when they touch the metal grid and fall into a collecting tray underneath.

Electrically operated fly-killer

COCKROACHES

There are many different types of cockroach of varying sizes but only two are commonly found in the UK: the German cockroach and the oriental cockroach. The German cockroach is the smaller and is found in the kitchens of restaurants, hotels and industrial canteens. Typical hiding places are behind ovens and hot water pipes and around refrigerator motors. The larger oriental cockroach is usually found in the cooler and less humid parts of buildings such as basements, cellars and store rooms.

Cockroaches spread the bacteria that cause food poisoning and also those that cause dysentery and typhoid.

Their presence is not always detected at an early stage because they hide in crevices and cavities in the daytime and emerge to feed only at night. As they move around the kitchen in search of food they contaminate work surfaces, utensils, equipment and any uncovered food with pathogenic bacteria from their droppings and bodies.

An infestation by cockroaches can be recognised by their droppings and a characteristic and very unpleasant smell. It can be treated with insecticides but expert advice must be sought about their use in food premises. Several treatments will be necessary because the eggs of the cockroach are protected by a capsule and do not hatch out for several months.

Oriental cockroach
(actual size 22 mm)

German cockroach
(actual size 12 mm)

PHARAOH'S ANTS

Pharaoh's ants are small red-brown tropical ants. Infestations are found in warm, usually permanently heated premises, such as hospitals and bakeries. These ants carry many pathogenic bacteria including some capable of causing food poisoning. In hospitals, they are attracted to soiled dressings, toilets and drains and can therefore transmit many diseases. As with all pest infestations, professional advice must be sought as soon as an infestation is suspected.

BIRDS

The most common pest birds are sparrows, pigeons and starlings. They have been called 'flying mice' because their droppings, feathers and feet are heavily contaminated with food poisoning bacteria. Birds can be removed from food premises by encouraging them to eat food mixed with a narcotic drug that causes deep sleep. They can then be removed from the premises and destroyed humanely. If any protected bird takes the bait, it can be revived and released unaffected.

SUMMARY

1. Rats, mice, flies, cockroaches and Pharaoh's ants are the most common kitchen pests.
2. Pests carry bacteria in their intestines, on their bodies and feet and can contaminate food or work surfaces with their droppings or by walking over them.
3. If a pest infestation is suspected, expert advice must be sought.
4. Electrically operated fly killers are the most satisfactory way of destroying flies in the kitchen.

Chapter 18

Food Spoilage and Food Preservation

FOOD SPOILAGE

All foods deteriorate on keeping. Changes in taste, texture, appearance and smell occur, frequently making the food inedible. The aim of food preservation is to reduce the rate at which this deterioration takes place. Most food spoilage is caused either by enzymes present in the food itself, or by the growth of micro-organisms (bacteria, moulds or yeasts).

Enzymes

Immediately after slaughter or harvest, enzymes present in food start to break down the cell structure of the food. This process is known as autolysis. Autolysis causes a deterioration in the appearance and texture of the food and also makes the food more susceptible to attack by micro-organisms.

Microbial spoilage

Bacteria, moulds and yeasts are all capable of causing food spoilage when they grow and multiply in or on food. Spoilage bacteria are naturally present in foods such as milk and meat, yeasts are often present on fruit, and mould spores are present in the air and start to muliply when they land on food. The type of spoilage will depend on a number of factors related to the food.

1. **The pH of the food.** The pH scale expresses the acidity or alkalinity of a substance. Water is neutral and has a pH of 7. Acid substances have a pH of less than 7 and alkaline substances have a pH greater than 7. Most foods are slightly acid. Egg white and some foods made with flour are weak alkalis.

104

The pH scale

   Bacteria are more likely to spoil foods with a near neutral pH, for example milk, cream, meat.

   Moulds and yeasts are more likely to spoil foods with a low pH, for example tomatoes, citrus fruits, fruit juices.

2. **The water activity of the food (Aw).** The water activity of a food is the amount of water that is available for microbial growth. The *Aw* of pure water is 1. Foods with plenty of available water have a high *Aw* (just less than 1). Foods with a high concentration of salt or sugar have a low *Aw* because the salt or sugar absorbs moisture and makes it unavailable for microbial growth.

    Bacteria are more likely to spoil foods with a high *Aw*, for example milk, meat, eggs, fish.

    Moulds are more likely to spoil foods with a lower *Aw*, for example bread, cheese, jam, cakes.

3. **The composition of the food.** Bacteria are more likely to spoil foods that are high in protein. Protein breakdown caused by bacteria results in the familiar unpleasant smells and tastes associated with 'off' meat, or 'bad' eggs. Bacteria, moulds and yeasts use carbohydrates present in the food as a source of energy. As they multiply they produce acids, alcohols and gases that make the food taste sour, alcoholic or bubbly.

FOOD PRESERVATION

In order to preserve food it is necessary to either destroy the micro-organisms that are present on or in the food, or to inhibit their growth in some way.

   The preservation methods used fall into the following groups.

1. Low temperature storage, for example refrigeration, freezing.

2. Use of high temperatures, for example cooking, pasteurisation and sterilisation (including canning).

3. Dehydration, for example drying, smoking, use of salt and sugar.

4. Use of chemical preservatives.

5. Vacuum packing.

6. Controlled atmosphere packaging.

7. Irradiation.

LOW TEMPERATURE STORAGE

Low temperature preservation of food can be either short term (refrigeration), or long term (freezing).

Refrigeration

The correct running temperature of a refrigerator is 1–4 °C. At this temperature most pathogens will not grow, but *Listeria* (see page 121) and *Yersinia* (see page 123) are exceptions. These bacteria will grow slowly at refrigeration temperatures and are found in a wide variety of foods. It is therefore important to observe the 'use-by' dates on all foods. Many spoilage bacteria grow slowly at refrigeration temperatures and hence the flavour, taste and texture of food stored in a refrigerator will deteriorate, but not as quickly as it would do at room temperature.

Freezing

The correct running temperature of a domestic freezer is −18 °C. Micro-organisms will not grow at this temperature, though many will remain dormant. Enzymatic changes do take place very slowly, giving some deterioration in the quality of the food when it is stored for a long period of time.

USE OF HIGH TEMPERATURES

The main reason for cooking food is to make it more palatable, but cooking also destroys many of the pathogenic bacteria and many of those that cause spoilage. Pasteurisation and sterilisation are the most common methods of preserving food by the application of heat. Pasteurisation is a short-term method of preservation and results in less change in the quality and nutritive value of the food than sterilisation, which is a long-term method and affects the quality and nutritive value of the food to a greater extent.

Pasteurisation

This mild heat process is designed to reduce the number of spoilage micro-organisms and destroy the pathogenic ones.

Milk was originally pasteurised to destroy the bacteria that cause tuberculosis. It is heated to 72 °C for 15 seconds and then cooled rapidly to below 10 °C. This process destroys *Salmonella* and *Campylobacter*, which may be present in raw milk, and also destroys some of the spoilage bacteria, so the milk will keep longer.

By law, liquid egg and ice cream mix must be pasteurised in order to destroy *Salmonella* and any other pathogens present. A number of different combinations of time and temperature are used to achieve pasteurisation of ice cream 65.6 °C for 30 minutes, 71.1 °C for 10 minutes, 79.4 °C for 15 seconds, followed by rapid cooling. A high temperature for a shorter time generally results in a better product with less loss of flavour. More heat is needed to pasteurise ice cream than milk because ice cream is rich in sugar and fat which give bacteria some protection.

Liquid egg is pasteurised at 64.4 °C for 2½ minutes and then cooled rapidly. The temperature at which it is pasteurised must be below 65 °C in order to prevent protein coagulation.

Sterilisation

This heat process is designed to kill all micro-organisms and their spores. Milk is sterilised by heating it in sealed bottles under pressure to 112 °C for 15 minutes.

Milk that has been sterilised has a 'cooked' flavour but it will keep for several years at room temperature.

Ultra-high-temperature (UHT) treatment

This heat process will destroy all micro-organisms but not all spores. The milk is heated to 132 °C for 1 second and then cooled rapidly and aseptically packed (a method of packing which does not allow the entry of any micro-organisms). UHT milk will keep for six months or more at room temperature and it has a better flavour than sterilised milk.

Canning

Canning is a widely used method of food preservation. The food is put in a metal can, sealed so that no further micro-organisms can enter the food, and then sterilised. The most important consideration is to ensure that any spores of *Clostridium botulinum* are destroyed, since this pathogen would thrive in canned foods because of the absence of oxygen (see page 122).

The time and temperature required to sterilise the food in the can depends on:

1. The size of the can.

2. The consistency of the food.

3. The pH of the food.

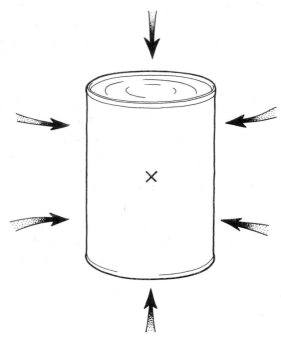

The heat has to penetrate to the food in the centre of the can.

Sufficient heat must be applied to sterilise the food in the centre of the can, allowing for the fact that heat has to penetrate from the outside to the centre. A large can of solid food, for example corned beef, will take longer to sterilise than a small can of liquid food, such as consommé. *Clostridium botulinum* and many other pathogens do not grow in very acid foods (pH less than 4.5), and hence acid foods require less heat treatment than near neutral foods in order to achieve sterilisation.

Aseptic canning

Aseptic canning is a variation on the standard canning process whereby the cans and the bulk product are sterilised separately and then filled in conditions that prevent the entry of any further micro-organisms. Aseptic canning is used for foods that are sensitive to heat, such as dairy custards and other milk products, which would be burnt at the surface in the standard canning process. It is a particularly useful method for large cans.

Pasteurised canned hams

Some catering-sized cans of ham are pasteurised rather than sterilised because the high temperatures required for sterilisation would cause shrinkage and loss of flavour. The saltiness of the product also helps to preserve it, but since some micro-organisms are present, pasteurised canned hams must be stored in a refrigerator. The manufacturer's storage instructions appear on the label and must be followed.

Spoilage of canned foods

Once a can has been opened the food in it must be treated as fresh food and stored in a refrigerator. Uneaten food must not be left in the can because it absorbs tin from the can, particularly if it is an acid food.

Unopened cans sometimes develop bulges at the ends due to gas produced inside the can. These cans are known as 'blown' cans and must not be used. The gas has probably been produced by bacteria, which means that either the can was under-sterilised or that it is a faulty can that has allowed bacteria to enter after sterilisation. Any other cans from the same batch (as indicated by the code on the end of the can), must not be used without discussing the problem with the manufacturer or an environmental health officer. Similarly, rusty or badly dented cans should not be used as it is possible that there will be a small opening somewhere in the can.

DEHYDRATION

Dehydration reduces the moisture content (Aw) of foods to levels at which micro-organisms cannot grow. Dehydrated foods are not sterile and bacteria can survive in them for many years. When dehydrated foods are reconstituted, any bacteria present will start to multiply. If the reconstituted food is not going to be used immediately, it should be refrigerated.

Smoking

Smoking is an ancient method of food preservation and now used mainly to give the food a characteristic flavour and texture rather than as a method of preservation. The drying effect on the surface of the food and several of the compounds in the smoke will inhibit the growth of some micro-organisms.

Salt and sugar

High concentrations of salt and sugar in food make the water in the food unavailable for microbial growth. Certain foods can therefore be preserved by the addition of salt or sugar. The preservative effect may be only partial and is often used with other preservative methods such as refrigeration.

Salt is used in the curing of foods such as pork and fish. The curing medium is a brine, containing sodium chloride (salt), sodium nitrate and sodium nitrite, in which the food is immersed or which is injected into the meat. Salted meat or fish has a characteristic flavour and colour.

Sugar is used mainly to preserve fruit in various forms such as jams, marmalades and crystallised fruits.

CHEMICAL PRESERVATIVES

Several chemicals are widely used in the preservation of food.

Acetic acid (vinegar) is used to preserve vegetables such as onions, cabbages, cauliflowers and gherkins, as well as for the manufacture of products such as chutney and salad cream. Adding vinegar lowers the pH of the food so that it is too acid for bacterial growth.

Making yoghurt is a traditional method of preserving milk. Bacteria that convert lactose to lactic acid are added to the milk to lower its pH.

Sulphur dioxide is added to many foods to help preserve them, including sausages, dried fruit, beer and wine. Sulphur dioxide in food is converted to sulphurous acid, which lowers the pH and hence has a preservative effect.

Sodium nitrate and sodium nitrite are used in the curing process and are also added to canned and vacuum-packed meats. Sodium nitrite very effectively inhibits the growth of *Clostridium botulinum*, but in recent years there has been some controversy over its use. It is thought that the ingestion of nitrites might possibly lead to the development of some types of cancer. It is however unlikely that the quantities used in food present any significant risk.

VACUUM PACKING

Vacuum packing foods stops the growth of aerobic micro-organisms such as moulds and some spoilage bacteria, but will not stop the growth of anaerobic bacteria. Vacuum packing hard cheeses prevents mould spoilage on the surface and the low moisture content of hard cheese inhibits bacterial growth. Vacuum packing will not inhibit the growth of *Clostridium botulinum*, and therefore when it is used with meats, where pathogenic bacteria including *Clostridium botulinum* may be present, it must be used in conjunction with other methods of preservation, for example refrigeration or the addition of nitrites.

CONTROLLED ATMOSPHERE PACKAGING

Carbon dioxide is sometimes used in conjunction with refrigeration to reduce the rate of spoilage of fresh meat, fruits, vegetables and eggs. The optimum concentration of carbon dioxide in the atmosphere varies depending on the type of food. Too much carbon dioxide in the atmosphere can cause tissue damage and produce 'off' flavours.

IRRADIATION

Irradiating food with gamma rays is an effective method of destroying both pathogenic and spoilage micro-organisms in foods such as raw chicken, fruit, vegetables, spices, shellfish and cereals. There is very little change, if any, in the taste or texture of the food as a result of irradiation. Irradiated food is considered to be perfectly safe to eat but there is a great reluctance by members of the public to accept foods that have been treated in this way. Any food that has been irradiated must be labelled accordingly.

Irradiation can be used to destroy *Salmonella* in animal feeds. If all feeds were treated in this way there would be a significant reduction in the number of animals carrying *Salmonella*. The expense of the process is the main prohibitive factor.

Chapter 19

Food Hygiene Legislation

FOOD SAFETY (GENERAL FOOD HYGIENE) REGULATIONS 1995

These regulations came into force on 15th September 1995 and are available from HMSO (SI 1995 No 1763). The Regulations aim to ensure that the same food hygiene rules are enforced in all European Union countries. Anyone who owns, manages or works in a food business must adhere to them. This includes people who transport, pack and store food, not just those who prepare it. All types of food businesses are included: anything from an expensive restaurant or large supermarket to a stall in a village hall or a vending machine.

The new regulations are in many ways similar to previous regulations, but rather than being simply a list of rules, a greater emphasis is put on proprietors identifying the food safety hazards likely to arise in their particular business and devising procedures to control these risks, ensuring that safe food is sold to the customer.

Requirements of the 1995 Food Safety Regulations

1. Rooms where food is prepared, treated or processed should:

    - be clean and maintained in good repair
    - have surface finishes which are easy to clean and, where necessary, disinfect
    - have an adequate supply of drinking water
    - have adequate facilities, including hot and cold water, for washing food and equipment
    - have adequate hand-washing facilities
    - have suitable controls in place to protect against pests
    - have adequate natural and/or artificial light
    - have sufficient natural and/or artificial ventilation. Filters must be accessible for cleaning
    - provide clean lavatories which do not lead directly into food rooms.

These basic minimum hygiene standards apply to all food businesses, but, for example, whether a surface is cleaned or disinfected, and how often, will depend on whether it is being used for the preparation of high-risk or low-risk foods.

2. All food handlers must maintain a high standard of personal hygiene. They should:

- wash hands frequently when handling food
- wear clean overalls
- never smoke whilst preparing food
- report to the manager any illnesses, particularly vomiting, diarrhoea and infected wounds.

It is expected that all food handlers will observe these rules but, for example, the frequency of hand-washing will vary depending on whether high-risk or low-risk foods are being handled.

FOOD SAFETY (TEMPERATURE CONTROL) REGULATIONS 1995

All food likely to support the growth of pathogenic bacteria or the formation of toxins must be stored at a temperature below 8 °C. If a food which would normally support the growth of micro-organisms is stored above 8 °C, the owner of the food business must be able to offer a scientific assessment (a microbiological analysis by a qualified scientist) of the safety of the food under the conditions in which it is stored. If the food is to be served hot it must be kept at a temperature of 63 °C or above. Food which is about to be served hot may be kept hot (but below 63 °C) for a maximum period of two hours. Food which is about to be served cold may be kept at a temperature above 8 °C for a maximum of four hours.

HAZARD ANALYSIS CRITICAL CONTROL POINT (HACCP)

A food hazard usually means the contamination of food by pathogenic bacteria, chemicals or other foreign materials. Every food business will have different hazards, depending on the types of food sold and the method of preparation.

Food businesses can satisfy themselves that their product is safe by setting up an HACCP team to identify the hazards and the points in the production process where they are most likely to occur (critical points). When this has been done it is possible to draw up a list of checks to be performed and specify who is to do the checks and at what intervals, in order to control the hazard.

For example, in the preparation and cooking of chicken for serving cold with salad, the food hazards most likely to occur are the growth of pathogenic micro-organisms due to poor temperature control and cross-contamination to or from other foods.

Step	Points to be considered
Purchase and delivery	Checks on the supplier
	Check on temperature and condition on delivery
Storage	Correct storage temperature?
	Can cross-contamination occur?
	Stock rotation?
Preparation	Length of time at room temperature?
	Cross-contamination?
	Cleaning of surfaces after preparation?
Cooking	Adequate cooking through to the centre of the chicken?
Cooling	Length of time at room temperature?
	Is refrigeration space available?
	Cross-contamination
Service	Length of time on display at room temperature

The 1995 Food Safety Regulations do not demand a fully documented HACCP but the proprietor has a legal obligation to establish a system and keep it under review. An outline of the checks in place for each process in the business would be useful to show an environmental health officer during an inspection and may be very important in establishing a defence of due diligence if necessary (see page 118).

Training

The Food Safety Regulations 1995 put the responsibility for hygiene training of food handlers onto the owner of a food business. The extent of training will be different for each individual depending on the type of food they handle. Staff who handle high-risk foods will need more training than those who handle low-risk foods. Special arrangements will have to be made for those employees whose first language is not English.

Staff may be trained 'in-house' or alternatively they should attend a food hygiene training course. A list of organisations who run food hygiene courses at various levels is given at the end of the chapter.

It is useful to keep a record of training given to each member of staff which is signed by the person concerned.

FOOD SAFETY ACT 1990

This Act is concerned with the safety of food from farm production to the point when it is sold. It is an offence to sell or possess for sale food that:

- is unfit to eat either because it is contaminated with pathogenic micro-organisms or because it contains poisonous chemicals or foreign bodies
- has false or misleading labelling or advertisement.

Two important provisions of the Food Safety Act 1990 are:

1. *Registration of Premises* Food premises including mobile premises such as hamburger vans must be registered with their local district council at least 28 days before trading begins. This gives the Environmental Health Officer opportunity to inspect the premises and give Food Safety advice where necessary. There is no charge for registration.

2. *Emergency Closure* Environmental health officers are allowed to close premises without notice if there is an immediate danger to public health.

ENFORCEMENT OF LEGISLATION

Food hygiene legislation is enforced by the Local Authority through the work of environmental health officers and trading standards officers. Environmental health officers deal with hygiene of food premises and cases where food is contaminated with micro-organisms or for any other reason is unfit for human consumption. Trading standards officers deal with the labelling of food, its composition and most cases of chemical contamination. In Scotland and Northern Ireland all food law is enforced by the environmental health departments of district councils. Apart from enforcing legislation environmental health officers are willing to give advice and guidance on any matter relating to food hygiene.

Powers to deal with unsafe food

If a food business is suspected of selling food that does not comply with food safety requirements an environmental health officer is able to:

1. Enter the premises to investigate.

2. Inspect food and take samples for analysis.

3. Prohibit the sale of any suspect food until a sample has been analysed.

4. Remove the suspect food and ask a Justice of the Peace to condemn it.

If the sample is found to be satisfactory and the rest of the detained food has deteriorated whilst the sample was analysed, the owner is entitled to compensation.

Inspection of Premises

Environmental health officers inspect all food businesses on a regular basis and will make extra visits if there is any reason to suspect that premises or practices are unhygienic. The environmental health officer identifies the risks attached to each particular business and considers the effectiveness of the systems employed to control potential problems. It is useful to have a brief written explanation of the systems in place to show the environmental health officer (see HACCP, page 113).

The main points that the environmental health officer considers are as follows:

1. Are the premises clean and well maintained?

2. Are the premises large enough for the scale of operation?

3. Is there adequate refrigeration space?

4. Is the food storage area adequate?

5. Is there an adequate number of sinks and wash hand basins?

6. Are the premises well lit and ventilated?

7. Are all the work surfaces clean and of suitable material?

8. Are all the utensils and equipment clean?

9. Are the methods of refuse disposal suitable?

10. Are there any signs of pest infestation?

11. Are the toilet facilities clean?

12. Is there a cleaning schedule in operation?

Do the staff:

Keep and prepare raw and cooked food separately?
Handle food as little as possible?
Ensure food is kept cold (below 8 °C), or hot (above 63 °C)?
Wear clean washable overalls?

Are the staff aware that:

They should not smoke whilst in a food room?
They should report any illness, especially vomiting or diarrhoea?
They should cover cuts with a waterproof plaster?

After an inspection the environmental health officer might write informally to the proprietor of the business asking him to put right any problems which have come to light during the inspection. If the offences are more serious he may take one of the following actions:

1. Issue an **Improvement Notice**, which requests that certain measures are taken in order to comply with food hygiene legislation. A specified time limit is set for the improvements to be made. (This will be at least a fortnight.)

2. Prosecute the proprietor for a breach of the food hygiene regulations. If the court feels that public health is at risk it will impose a **Prohibition Order**, which closes all the business or the part of the business that does not comply with the regulations.

3. Issue an **Emergency Prohibition Notice**. If the offence imposes an immediate risk to health, the environmental health officer can close the premises immediately for three days by issuing an

Emergency Prohibition Notice. The matter is taken before a court within three days. If the court agrees that the offence poses an immediate risk to health it will issue an **Emergency Prohibition Order**, which keeps the premises closed until the necessary improvements have been made.

To lift a Prohibition Order or an Emergency Prohibition Order and re-open the premises the proprietor must apply to the environmental health officer for a **Certificate of Satisfaction**.

Food hygiene offences are usually brought to a Magistrates' Court, where the penalty for contravening the legislation is a maximum fine of £5000 for each offence and/or a prison sentence of up to six months. If the offence concerns false or misleading labelling or contamination, there is a maximum fine of £20 000 (Food Safety Act 1990). Food hygiene offences can be brought to a Crown Court. There is no maximum fine in a Crown Court and a prison sentence of up to two years may be imposed.

Due diligence defence

Every food handler is responsible for ensuring that the food he or she manufactures, transports, prepares or serves is safe to eat. If food is found to be unfit to eat, the person responsible will be prosecuted unless he can prove he took all reasonable precautions (exercised all due diligence) to avoid causing the offence. This defence can be established if a food handler can prove:

1. It is the fault of another person.

2. Someone he trusted should have carried out all necessary checks.

3. He had no reason to believe that his omission or action would amount to an offence.

A due diligence defence might be appropriate if, for example, a caterer was supplied with ready prepared meals which turned out to cause food poisoning. The caterer would have to prove that he had taken all reasonable precautions to avoid this situation by carrying out all necessary checks on the method of production and by obtaining details of storage and transportation temperatures of the food before delivery. Written records of the date and types of checks made would be very valuable in such a defence.

INVESTIGATION OF AN OUTBREAK OF FOOD POISONING

Any person who suspects that they are suffering from food poisoning should go to their doctor who is obliged to inform the local environmental health officer if he thinks his patient is suffering from food poisoning.

Outbreaks of food poisoning are investigated by the environmental health officer.

All patients are questioned about their symptoms, what food they have eaten in the last 48 hours and where it was eaten. Samples of their faeces are sent to a public health laboratory for bacteriological examination. If staphylococcal food poisoning is suspected, samples of vomit may be sent for analysis.

If most of the patients bought their food at a particular shop or restaurant, the environmental health officer will visit the premises and collect samples of any remaining suspect food.

A faecal sample will be taken from anyone who is in contact with food at the premises, and if staphylococcal infection is suspected, nose, throat and skin swabs will be taken. Working surfaces and equipment may also be swabbed. All the samples are sent to the public health laboratory where they are checked to see whether they carry bacteria identical to those isolated from the patient.

If the cause of the outbreak is discovered, appropriate action will be taken to ensure that no further outbreaks occur. Food handlers who are suffering from the same illness will be excluded from work. They may return to work 48 hours after the vomiting and diarrhoea have ceased provided no medication is being taken to control the symptoms. If the food handler is infected with S. typhi or S. paratyphi, exclusion from work continues until six consecutive negative stool samples taken at 14-day intervals are obtained. The local authority will pay the food handler's wages for the period he is excluded from work but he will, however, be prosecuted if he returns to work during that period. If inadequate temperature control or cross-contamination is responsible for the outbreak of food poisoning, advice is given about storage and preparation of high-risk foods.

ORGANISATIONS RUNNING FOOD HYGIENE TRAINING COURSES

Chartered Institute of Environmental Health
Tel: 0171-928 6006

Royal Institute of Public Health and Hygiene
Tel: 0171-580 2731

Royal Society of Health
Tel: 0171-630 0121

Society of Food Hygiene Technology
Tel: 01590 671979

Appendix

Further Causes of Food Poisoning and Food-Borne Diseases

A few outbreaks of food poisoning are recorded each year which are attributed to causes other than those already described.

Listeria monocytogenes

Cases of illness attributed to *Listeria monocytogenes* are relatively rare, but these bacteria have attracted a lot of media attention, partly because the illness they cause can be serious or even fatal and partly because they are one of the few types of pathogenic bacteria that can grow at refrigeration temperatures.

Listeria monocytogenes is found widely distributed in the environment and is present in the intestines of many domestic and wild animals including chickens, sheep and cattle. The bacteria can be passed into the milk of infected animals.

The vast majority of people who eat food contaminated with *Listeria monocytogenes* will be unaffected or may at worst have a mild fever for a short time. However, two groups of people are particularly at risk of severe illness: pregnant women and sick people whose illness or treatment affects their immune system. Listeriosis in pregnant women can cause miscarriage or result in a still birth. In very young babies and in immunosuppressed patients, listeriosis gives rise to meningitis and septicaemia.

Foods that have frequently been found to contain *Listeria* and that should therefore be avoided by the two vulnerable groups include soft ripened cheeses, for example Brie and Camembert, pâté, cook-chill meals, coleslaw and other pre-packed salads in dressings, salami and continental sausages.

Clostridium botulinum

Food poisoning by *Clostridium botulinum* is very rare in the UK, but because many of the cases that occur are fatal, great efforts are made to avoid causing this type of food poisoning.

Clostridium botulinum causes toxic food poisoning. The toxin is produced by the bacteria when they are growing in food under strictly anaerobic conditions (a complete absence of oxygen), for example in canned food. The toxin is a highly poisonous substance and people have died after eating only a mouthful of infected food. The symptoms are giddiness, double vision, headache, nausea and vomiting. The central nervous system is affected and paralysis of the respiratory tract is the usual cause of death.

Clostridium botulinum is found in soil and therefore on vegetables. It is also found in fish caught in some areas, notably the waters around Japan. It can produce a spore which will survive ordinary cooking methods but the toxin produced by it is not heat resistant and will usually be destroyed by boiling for a few minutes.

Most cases of botulism (food poisoning caused by *C. botulinum*) have occurred after eating under-sterilised canned food or food in faulty cans which has been contaminated after sterilisation. Food manufacturers take great care that all *C. botulinum* spores are destroyed in processing and only very rarely have commercially canned foods been the cause of this type of food poisoning. In the United States of America, some people can their own vegetables and this has sometimes caused botulism. A Japanese delicacy, of raw fermented fish, has also caused outbreaks of botulism.

Vibrio parahaemolyticus

Vibrio parahaemolyticus is a comma-shaped bacterium. It is a common contaminant of fish and shellfish in tropical and subtropical waters. The few outbreaks of *V. parahaemolyticus* food poisoning which occur in the United Kingdom are usually traced to the consumption of imported seafood which has been contaminated after cooking (*V. parahaemolyticus* is sensitive to heat) and has been left unrefrigerated for some time.

The symptoms which usually occur between 12 and 18 hours after eating the contaminated food are abdominal pain and profuse diarrhoea often with vomiting and fever. The illness lasts from 2 to 5 days.

Although rare in Britain, *V. parahaemolyticus* is one of the most common causes of food poisoning in Japan.

Escherichia coli

Escherichia coli is a small rod-shaped bacterium. It is present in the intestinal tract of healthy people and is not normally pathogenic, but there are a few serotypes which are capable of causing diarrhoea in young children (usually under two years old). Adults are very rarely affected except when travelling abroad. 'Traveller's diarrohea' is usually caused by a serotype of *E. coli* which is not found in the traveller's home country but may be widespread in the foreign country.

The symptoms which usually occur between 12 and 24 hours after eating the contaminated food are abdominal pain, fever, diarrhoea and sometimes vomiting. The illness lasts from 1–5 days.

E. coli is used as an indicator organism in food analysis. The presence of *E. coli* in food suggests that the food has at some stage been contaminated from a faecal source and therefore implies that there is a potential risk of the presence of more harmful intestinal organisms such as *Salmonella.*

Yersinia enterocolytica

Yersinia enterocolytica is a rod-shaped bacterium that has been isolated from many foods, including raw milk, ice cream, mussels, canned and vacuum-packed meat, prawns and beefburgers. It can grow slowly at temperatures as low as 1–3 °C. Cells grown at low temperatures are more virulent than those grown at higher temperatures. The main symptom which occurs 24–36 hours after consumption of the infected food, is diarrhoea, sometimes accompanied by abdominal pains, fever and vomiting. The number of reported cases of this type of food poisoning is very low.

Scombrotoxic fish poisoning

Scombrotoxic fish poisoning was first reported in the United Kingdom in 1976 and since then there have been several incidents as a result of the consumption of mackerel, tuna, sardines or pilchards. These fish are rich in the amino acid histidine which is converted to histamine by spoilage bacteria present in the fish. Histamine combines with another substance to form a toxin. Lengthy periods of unrefrigerated storage allow the formation of sufficient toxin in the flesh of the fish to cause symptoms similar to an allergic reaction. The symptoms occur between 15 minutes and 3 hours after eating the fish and include a burning sensation in the mouth and throat, puffiness around the eyes, swelling of the lips, tongue and gums, urticaria, headache, nausea, vomiting and diarrhoea. They last for 8 to 12 hours. The toxin is not easily destroyed by heat, and canned fish can also cause scombrotoxic fish poisoning.

Paralytic shellfish poisoning

Paralytic shellfish poisoning (PSP) occurs only rarely in the United Kingdom but it is a serious and sometimes fatal type of food poisoning. It can occur following the consumption of mussels or oysters which have been feeding on a certain type of toxic plankton resulting in the accumulation of toxins in the flesh of the fish.

Symptoms occur between ½ and 3 hours after eating the fish and include a tingling of the tongue and mouth which spreads to the neck, fingers and toes and occasionally progresses to paralysis. PSP is most likely to occur in exceptionally warm weather. A large outbreak occurred in 1968 involving mussels, and since then annual monitoring of the toxin levels in mussels has taken place.

Brucellosis and tuberculosis

These two diseases are usually spread by contaminated milk. Since the introduction of pasteurisation of milk, they have become rare. Pasteurisation is a heating process which ensures that all pathogenic bacteria are destroyed although some spoilage bacteria and other non-pathogenic bacteria may remain alive.

Brucellosis (Undulant fever) is caused by a bacterium called *Brucella abortus*.

Incubation period	5–21 days
Symptoms	Variable but usually pain in muscles and joints and a fever. The disease is rarely fatal but can give rise to prolonged ill health.

Tuberculosis is caused by a species of the genus *Mycobacterium*.

Incubation period	4–6 weeks
Symptoms	The bovine type affects the bones, lymph nodes and intestines and is usually caused by drinking unpasteurised milk from infected cattle. The other type affects the lungs and is airborne. Both types of tuberculosis, though rare now, were common diseases in the early part of this century.

Control of brucellosis and tuberculosis.

1. Cattle herds are now checked regularly to ensure that they are free from these diseases. Infected animals are slaughtered.

2. Pasteurisation of milk.

VIRAL FOOD-BORNE DISEASES

Two groups of viruses frequently cause diarrhoea and vomiting: *rotaviruses* and *Norwalk-like viruses (NLV)*. Viruses cannot multiply in food and the food involved is merely a means of transport of the virus. *Rotaviruses* affect young children causing severe diarrhoea and vomiting and sometimes dehydration. The incubation period is usually four days and the illness may last up to a week. Adults are not affected but often transfer the disease by inadequate hand-washing between changing nappies and handling food or feeding bottles.

Norwalk-like viruses cause winter vomiting disease, which affects adults and children. The incubation period is 24–48 hours and the illness rarely lasts more than 48 hours. The symptoms are nausea and vomiting. Abdominal pain, diarrhoea and fever may also be present. Winter vomiting disease is transferred by the faecal oral route from infected food handlers and also by shellfish collected from sewage-polluted water.

Hepatitis

The strict meaning of hepatitis is inflamed liver. There are two types of viral hepatitis: hepatitis A and hepatitis B. Hepatitis A (also called infective hepatitis) is transmitted by food. Hepatitis B can only be transmitted directly from blood to blood.

Hepatitis A: accounts for the majority of cases. It is more likely to be contracted in Middle or Far Eastern countries than in the UK. The incubation period is long (about 2–7 weeks) and the symptoms are fever, nausea, abdominal pain and, later, jaundice. The 'duration' of the illness can be anything from a week to several months and the severity of the symptoms varies considerably.

The virus is spread by the faecal–oral route and so food can be contaminated by a food handler with poor hygiene standards who is a carrier of the virus. Many outbreaks are associated with shellfish collected from sewage-contaminated waters.

PROTOZOAL FOOD-BORNE DISEASES

Protozoa are single-celled micro-organisms. They live in an aqueous environment, e.g. soil saturated with water, ponds, ditches, rivers and the sea. The majority are harmless but a few are pathogenic to humans.

Giardiasis

Giardiasis is caused by the protozoan *Giardia lamblia*. The illness occurs world-wide but is more common in areas of poor sanitation where water has been contaminated with sewage. Giardiasis is spread by the faecal-oral route and outbreaks in the UK are often traced to food handlers returning from abroad.

The incubation period is 1-4 weeks and the predominant symptom is profuse watery diarrhoea often accompanied by abdominal pain and nausea. The severity of the symptoms varies considerably. *Giardia lamblia* is not heat-resistant and is easily killed by boiling.

Cryptosporidiosis

The protozoan *Cryptosporidium* is found in water contaminated with sewage. Cryptosporidiosis is widespread in animals and a common cause of diarrhoea in calves. The infection can be spread in humans by the faecal-oral route or directly from animals to humans. Milk, water and food have also been implicated. *Cryptosporidium* can survive the pasteurisation process and may survive some water treatment processes. The main symptoms are vomiting, diarrhoea, abdominal pain and fever which last for about 10 days.

Amoebic dysentery

Amoebic dysentery is caused by the protozoan *Entamoeba hystolytica*. The disease is spread by the faecal-oral route from infected individuals or from contaminated water or food. The incubation period is usually 3-4 weeks and the main symptoms are abdominal pain and diarrhoea.

Although rare in Europe it is endemic in some tropical countries particularly where sanitation and hygiene are primitive.

PARASITIC WORMS

Tapeworms

Tapeworm infestations have been more or less eliminated in the UK but are still common in tropical countries. The reported cases in the UK have almost always been acquired abroad.

Tapeworms can be found in cattle and pigs and the eggs produced by them are present in the animal's faeces. Ingested tapeworm eggs hatch into larvae (little grubs) which burrow through the intestinal wall to the bloodstream and are carried to the muscle of the animal where they form cysts. The cysts are easily visible in meat, giving it a spotted appearance. If the meat is eaten raw or undercooked, the cyst survives and starts to grow into an adult tapeworm. Adult tapeworms can be treated easily but the larvae can form cysts in the muscle or soft tissue of humans causing serious illness.

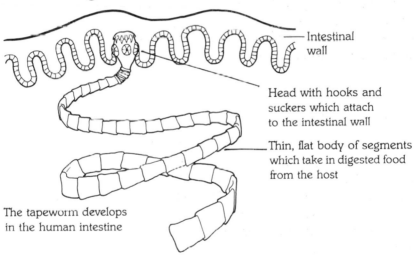

Intestinal wall

Head with hooks and suckers which attach to the intestinal wall

Thin, flat body of segments which take in digested food from the host

The tapeworm develops in the human intestine

Trichinosis

Trichinosis is caused by a very small worm, *Trichinella spiralis*. The disease is transmitted by pork. The life cycle is similar to that of tapeworms but the cysts are too small to be seen in the meat. The last outbreak of Trichinosis in the UK was in 1955. The few reported cases since then have been acquired abroad.

When travelling abroad, the standard hygiene precautions of not eating unwashed salad, vegetables or fruit, or undercooked or raw meat, and not drinking untreated water should protect a traveller from worm infestations.

Examination Questions

Chapter 1
1. Are all bacteria harmful? Describe the effects which different types of bacteria have on food.

Chapter 2
1. What are the four requirements for bacterial growth? Write a short paragraph about each one.
2. Write notes on:
   (a) Spores.
   (b) Foods which are susceptible to bacterial growth.
   (c) Anaerobes.
3. Describe the conditions which make bacteria dormant.

Chapter 3
1. Write notes on:
   (a) Incubation periods for bacterial food poisoning.
   (b) Chemical food poisoning.
   (c) Vegetable food poisoning.
   (d) Viral food poisoning.

Chapter 4
1. Explain what is meant by cross-contamination. If you owned a butcher's shop what advice would you give to your staff to prevent this occurring?
2. In what ways are pathogenic bacteria spread to food?
3. What are (a) healthy carriers and (b) convalescent carriers? What could be the result of a 'carrier' working in a food preparation area?

Chapter 5
1. What precautions would you take when preparing food to prevent *Salmonella* food poisoning arising?
2. Which bacterium causes the majority of food poisoning outbreaks? How is it usually spread into foods?

Chapter 6
1. If you were in charge of preparing sandwiches for a self-service counter, what precautions would you take to ensure that food poisoning due to *Staphylococcus aureus* did not occur?
2. Explain why a food can cause bacterial food poisoning even if there are no live bacteria in it?

Chapter 7
1. Why is the bacterium *Clostridium perfringens* particularly difficult to destroy? What precautions can you take to prevent this type of food poisoning occurring?
2. How is *Clostridium perfringens* usually brought into the kitchen? What would be a typical chain of events leading to this type of food poisoning?

Chapter 8
1. Why is it particularly important that meat products and rice should not be reheated more than once?

Chapter 9
1. Explain what is meant by 'bacterial food-borne diseases'. How do these differ from food poisoning?

Chapter 10
1. Why is it particularly important to maintain a high standard of personal hygiene when preparing food?
2. Write what you know about the following:
   (a) The hand-washing facilities which must, by law, be provided for food handlers.
   (b) The advantages and disadvantages of the various methods of hand-drying.
   (c) The occasions when hands must be washed.

Chapter 11
1. Give reasons for the following statements:
   (a) 'Thaw frozen meat completely before cooking.'
   (b) 'Keep food either very hot or very cold.'
2. Describe the common faults in food preparation which frequently contribute to outbreaks of food poisoning.

Chapter 12
1. Which foods should always be stored in a refrigerator and why? How would you position the foods you have mentioned in the refrigerator?
2. Why are refrigerators important in the prevention of food poisoning? How can you ensure that the temperature of the refrigerator is maintained?
3. Why can food be kept for a longer period of time in a freezer than in a refrigerator? What would you do if your freezer broke down?

4. Write a short description of the cook-chill and cook-freeze methods of food preparation.

Chapter 13
1. What types of food do not normally support the growth of food poisoning bacteria? In each case explain briefly why this is so.
2. Made-up meat dishes are frequently a cause of food poisoning. Give reasons for this.
3. Make a list of milk and dairy products which are often used in the kitchen and give reasons why some of them may cause food poisoning and others normally do not.

Chapter 14
1. What are the principal reasons for the increase in the number of outbreaks of food poisoning in the UK?
2. Why are there more outbreaks of food poisoning during the summer months than during the winter months?

Chapter 15
1. In a restaurant serving 100 meals each evening, describe how you would organise the washing-up if you did not have a dish-washing machine.
2. Describe the different functions of detergents and disinfectants and their importance in preventing food poisoning.

Chapter 16
1. If you were asked to plan a new kitchen what points regarding the design and layout would you consider important?
2. Why is efficient waste disposal important in the prevention of food poisoning?

Chapter 17
1. What indications might there be of an infestation by rats or mice? What action would you take?
2. What are the most common kitchen pests? How can they cause food poisoning?
3. What steps can you take to reduce the risk of an infestation of pests in your food premises?

Chapter 18
1. What are the main causes of food spoilage and what factors related to the food will determine the type of spoilage?
2. Give details of the main methods of food preservation.

Chapter 19
1. Give a brief summary of The Food Safety Regulations 1995 under the following headings:
   (a) Premises.
   (b) Personal hygiene.
   (c) Temperature control of food.
2. An outbreak of food poisoning has occurred among school children. How would this outbreak be investigated?
3. What powers does the Food Safety Act 1990 give to an environmental health officer inspecting food premises?

General
1. 'Food poisoning will occur only if food is prepared in dirty premises.' Discuss this statement.
2. What would you include in a lecture on food hygiene to a group of hospital caterers?
3. Which of the following foods particularly favour the growth of food poisoning bacteria and which rarely do? Explain why.
   (a) A 'rare' steak.
   (b) Stuffed, rolled breast of lamb.
   (c) Fried rice.
   (d) A cheddar cheese sandwich.
4. What hand-washing facilities should be provided in food premises and why?
5. What are the reasons for not allowing pets into food premises?
6. Write notes on three of the following:
   (a) Methods of waste disposal.
   (b) Materials suitable for use as working surfaces.
   (c) Lighting and ventilation in kitchens.
   (d) Keeping the kitchen free of flies.
7. 'Provided that food is hot, it is safe to eat.' Discuss this statement.
8. Which raw foods frequently carry food poisoning bacteria? How can cross–contamination be prevented?
9. Write briefly about three bacteria which commonly cause food poisoning in Britain.
10. Write notes on four of the following:
    (a) *Vibrio cholerae.*
    (b) *Clostridium botulinum.*
    (c) *Salmonella typhi.*
    (d) *Campylobacter.*
    (e) *Shigella.*

11. You have decided to go on a day trip in the car with some friends. You will be leaving early in the morning, stopping for lunch at a restaurant and packing a picnic tea. When deciding what to take, what points would you bear in mind to prevent food poisoning occurring?

12. Describe the food hygiene precautions you would take if organising a wedding reception for one hundred people to be held under canvas in June.

Royal Society of Health examination questions

Taken from the RSH certificate examination in the hygiene of food retailing and catering.

1. List three ways in which food may become contaminated in a kitchen.

2. List the three main conditions necessary for encouraging the growth of bacteria in foods.

3. Does the appearance of food normally indicate the presence of food poisoning organisms?

4. What food poisoning organism is frequently associated with pre-cooked meat meals?

5. (a) Above what temperature should foods that are to be kept hot be stored?
    (b) Below what temperature should foods that are to be kept cold be stored?

6. What should a food handler do in the following circumstances:
    (a) If a finger is cut.
    (b) If suffering from sickness and diarrhoea?

7. Why should poultry be defrosted before cooking?

8. What do you understand by the term 'incubation period' with respect to food poisoning?

9. State precisely the meaning of cross-contamination.

10. If a member of the public became ill with acute vomiting shortly after consuming a Chinese meal containing rice, which food poisoning organism would you suspect?

11. Make a list of high-risk foods.

12. Give two reasons why a kitchen must be well ventilated.

13. What action could an environmental health officer take if he/she found premises which were so dirty as to be a risk to public health?

14. What would lead you to suspect that your premises were infested with rats?
15. Briefly describe the 'two-sink system' of dish-washing.
16. What is a tap proportioner?
17. What is the title of the legislation which regulates hygiene in all food premises?
18. What is a pathogen?
19. What is a carrier?
20. What comments can you make on the practice of placing the 'sweets' trolley in a restaurant dining room throughout the evening?
21. State three important rules which should always be remembered when using a refrigerator.
22. Which harmful bacteria are most likely to be transferred to food by a food handler who bites his/her finger nails?
23. Why is it considered unwise to stuff a chicken before it is cooked?
24. Why are rolled joints of meat less safe than solid joints of meat?
25. What are the three most important precautions to undertake when preparing poultry in a kitchen?
26. Name two diseases other than food poisoning that may be transmitted by food.
27. What is the recognised maximum keeping time for 'cook-chill' foods?
28. Statistics show that food poisoning is on the increase. Give two causes for this increase.
29. Frozen food manufacturers use star markings on packages to provide the consumer and others with storage life information. Give the storage life and equivalent temperature for the following:
    (a) one star.
    (b) two stars.
    (c) three stars.
30. If frozen food defrosts, is it good practice to refreeze it?

GCE Advanced level domestic science and home economics examination questions

1. What is food poisoning and how is it caused? When does food poisoning constitute a real danger to life?
   Consider the implications of a chef with a heavy cold preparing dishes for the sweet trolley.
   (The Associated Examining Board)

2. Describe the ways in which bacterial food poisoning may be
    caused. Comment on the fact that food handlers need to use all
    the knowledge they can acquire to help reduce the incidence of
    food poisoning.
    (The Associated Examining Board)
3. Compare the properties of the materials used to make the follow-
    ing and say how those properties affect the use and care of the
    equipment in each case.
    (a) An enamelled sink and a stainless-steel sink.
    (b) A wooden chopping board and a laminated plastic chopping
        board.
    (c) Vinyl floor tiles and quarry tiles in an institutional kitchen.
    What general principles of design should be incorporated in
    equipment in order to make its use and cleaning as easy and as
    effective as possible?
    Evaluate the contribution to efficient and safe working that good
    lighting and ventilation systems can make in a canteen kitchen.
    (The Associated Examining Board)
4. Begin each sentence with the name of the appropriate micro-
    organism:
    (a) _____ is found in the nasal cavity of many individuals
        and can cause food poisoning.
    (b) _____ survives inadequate canning or bottling and may
        cause death.
    (c) _____ exists in poultry and survives inadequate cooking
        to cause food poisoning.
    (University of London)
5. Name three of the chief micro-organisms responsible for out-
    breaks of food poisoning and suggest two potential sources of
    each.
    (University of London)
6. (a) Discuss the link between micro-organisms and food-borne
        illnesses.
    (b) Assess the importance of hygiene in the home in the
        prevention of these illnesses.
        (Joint Matriculation Board)

Index

135